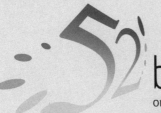

brilliantideas
one good idea can change your life...

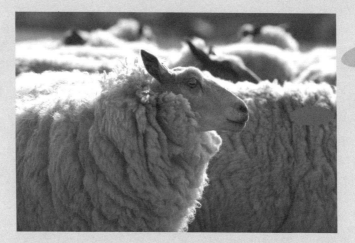

Sleep deep

Wake refreshed day after day

Karen Williamson

CAREFUL NOW

We know you're responsible and perfectly capable of using the information in this book wisely. That said, any advice given is not a substitute for medical advice – so consult your doctor or healthcare provider before making any changes to your diet and exercise regime or if you start taking supplements – particularly if you're on medication, you're very unfit or you're pregnant. Yes, we checked the facts, but teams of eager scientists in laboratories around the world are constantly updating and reassessing their research. So the facts might change. We like you and hope you're soon sleeping soundly every night, but we're not going to come around and tuck you in – because how well you sleep is ultimately up to you.

First published in 2005 by
The Infinite Ideas Company Limited
36 St Giles
Oxford, OX1 3LD
United Kingdom
www.infideas.com

A CIP catalogue record for this book is available from the British Library

ISBN 1-904902-49-9

Brand and product names are trademarks or registered trademarks of their respective owners.

Designed by Baseline Arts Ltd, Oxford
Typeset by Sparks, Oxford
Printed by TJ International, Cornwall

Brilliant ideas

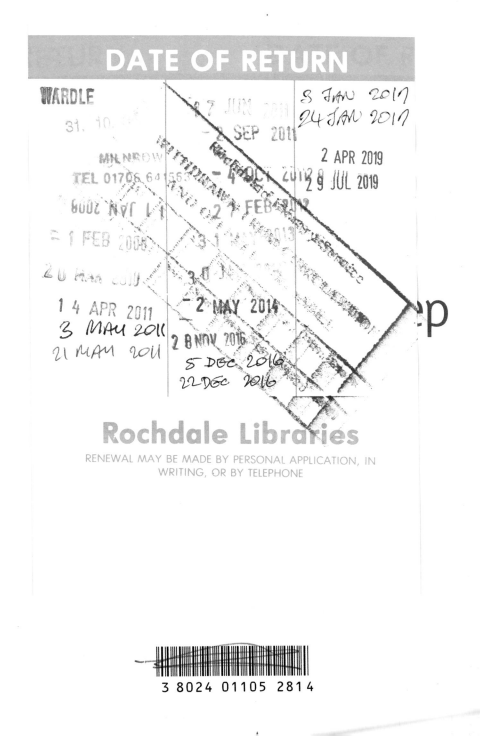

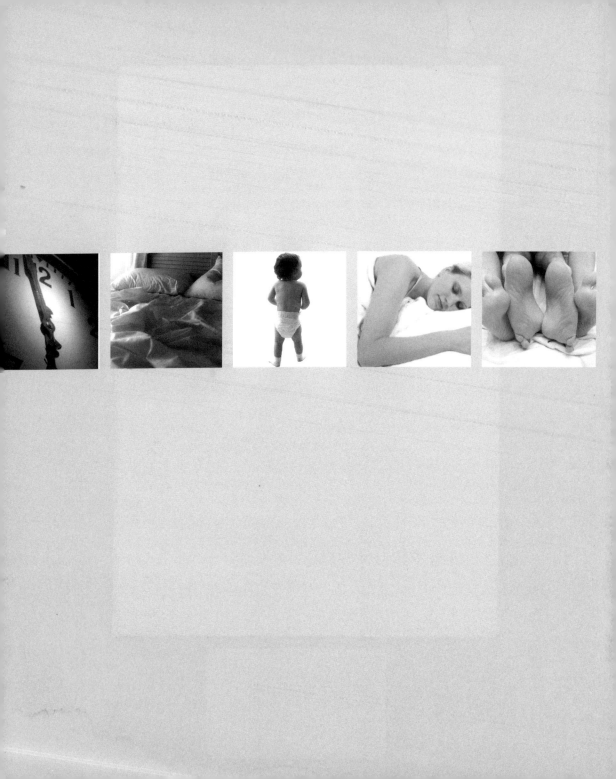

Brilliant features

Each chapter of this book is designed to provide you with an inspirational idea that you can read quickly and put into practice straight away.

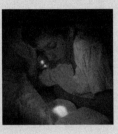

Throughout you'll find four features that will help you get right to the heart of the idea:

- *Here's an idea for you ...* Take it on board and give it a go – right here, right now. Get an idea of how well you're doing so far.

- *Try another idea ...* If this idea looks like a life-changer then there's no time to lose. *Try another idea ...* will point you straight to a related tip to enhance and expand on the first.

- *Defining idea ...* Words of wisdom from masters and mistresses of the art, plus some interesting hangers-on.

- *How did it go?* If at first you do succeed, try to hide your amazement. If, on the other hand, you don't, then this is where you'll find a Q and A that highlights common problems and how to get over them.

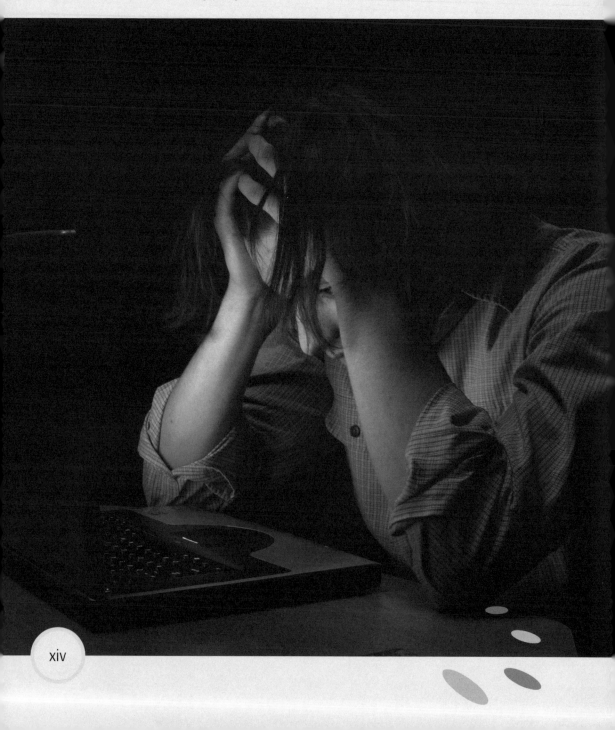

Introduction

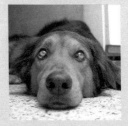

You don't really question sleep until you're not getting enough. And it's only when symptoms spiral out of control that you think about doing anything. Suddenly you're falling asleep during conversations, you're unable to concentrate on anything longer than a TV ad break, you can't be bothered to socialise any more and it's the fourth time this week you've put the tea bag in cold water. Even then, it often takes a comment from someone – 'Gosh you've been looking tired lately', 'You're not as lively as you used to be' or 'If you don't do something about your snoring, I'm going to leave you' – before you actually decide to take action.

I've seen many parents reduced to shadows of their former selves after extended periods of sleep deprivation. Those in top decision-making jobs become unable to decide what to have for breakfast, reduced to tears if they find the cornflakes packet empty. Fiercely bright men and women armed with first class degrees unable to recall their own middle names. For the most part however, parents get through this bleak period and find their brains, memory and dignity (well, brains and memory anyway) intact.

By far the biggest cause of insomnia, however, is stress. Study after study shows that we've got too much on our plate nowadays. We're working longer hours and there's more demanded of us at work. The constant threat of redundancy that most of us are under means that we're not even being rewarded for all our efforts. Then there's money – you can't even begin to think about how you're going to pay your £4000 credit card bill. It's not surprising panicky thoughts are keeping you up at night.

Chances are you're always on the go. It's very difficult to switch off from the world because there are no quiet times any more. You can pretty much do anything you want at any time of the day or night – from buying frozen peas to organising a bank loan. Then there's the overwhelming amount of choice which makes every decision you make increasingly difficult – from choosing a breakfast cereal to deciding which of the 268 shades of white to paint your downstairs toilet. At this rate, it's a wonder any of us get any sleep at all.

Many people I spoke to when writing this book had suffered insomnia for years, but had never done anything about it. They simply didn't know where to start and were unconvinced that anything could work. The fact is, there are some pretty straight-forward strategies to help you get the sleep you deserve. Just understanding what happens to your body while you sleep will help you work out the mechanisms behind your sleep problems – whether it's insomnia, nightmares, restless legs syndrome or sleep apnoea. And finding out about your body clock means you won't waste time trying out things that won't ever work. If you're a night owl, for instance, there's no point going to bed at 10p.m. – you'll be staring at the ceiling for 5 hours, churning over your thoughts. By the time you're ready to drop off, you'll have convinced yourself that you're going to get the sack, die horribly on your cycle ride to work, be abandoned by your partner or be told that the mole you've been thinking about is definitely cancerous.

The key to solving your sleep problem is finding the cause – be it stress, bad diet, a noisy bedroom environment – and being persistent. That means not giving up if the first thing you try doesn't work. If you need to relax, and yoga doesn't do it for you, try another relaxation technique. Maybe music or mental tricks will suit you better. Look at your diet and lifestyle too – particularly if you're regularly having late night takea-ways. The wrong foods, for instance, can lead to snoring, nightmares and disrupted and disturbed sleep and can make restless legs syndrome worse. And exercise helps by tackling stress and making you feel good about yourself as well as regulating your body clock and helping trigger all those sleep hormones at the right time. I've come up with a huge selection of tried-and-tested solutions so I guarantee you won't run out of things to do – from changing your bedtime routine and visualisation tricks to decluttering your bedroom and performing wake-me-up morning stretches.

Try everything that takes your fancy, write down how well it worked, keep referring back to your notes and soon you should have a list of all those changes you've made that do the trick. It may take one week or it may take a few months. But don't give up. Before you know it, you'll be sleeping soundly every night, waking up in a great mood and managing to stay full awake during every conversation you have in the day.

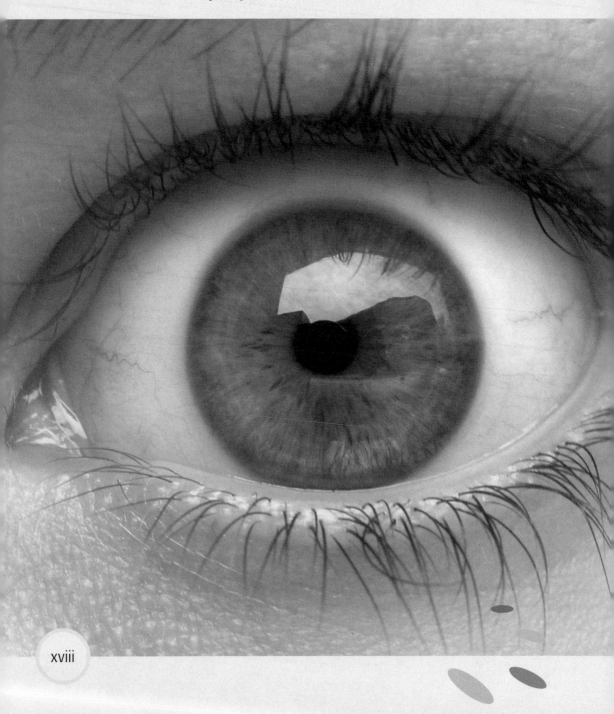

1

Eyes wide shut

We spend a third of our lives asleep – so what actually happens to our bodies when we're tucked up under the duvet?

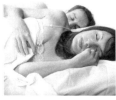

If you think sleep is when the body simply shuts down, you're much mistaken. Decades of tests involving wires, electrodes and imaginary sheep, have shown us just how complicated a process it is. You don't need a degree in human biology to understand it, but it helps …

While you're asleep your body produces a series of distinct brainwaves. They repeat themselves to form sleep cycles, each lasting around 60 minutes in babies and 90 minutes in adults. During a night, a normal sleeper can expect to go through 4–5 cycles. And each sleep cycle goes through five stages of sleep.

The body is thought to repair and regenerate itself in the first four stages of sleep – commonly known as non-REM sleep (NREM). Stage 5, REM (rapid eye-movement) sleep, is where the fun starts: learning is processed as the brain sorts out and makes

Here's an idea for you...

Want to see if your child, dog or partner is dreaming? When they're asleep, look at their eyes – you'll be able to detect the movement of their eyeballs through their eyelids. This means they're in REM sleep – the time they're most likely to dream.

sense of the events of the day – the argument you had with your boss, why you lost at squash and why you bought that glow-in-the-dark razor for your father. You are also most likely to dream.

To make it clearer, I'll take you through a night when you're having no trouble with your sleep. Before falling asleep, you close your eyes, your body relaxes and your brainwaves change from the rapid beta waves to slower, sleepier alpha waves. It's similar to the feeling you get when you keep nodding off while trying to read *War and Peace.* Then you get to:

- *Stage 1: light sleep.* Heart rate and body temperature drop and brainwaves slow down even more. It lasts a few minutes and you can easily be woken up during this stage. Ever been woken up by your own snoring on the bus and had to get off three stops early to escape public humiliation? Yes? Well you were probably in light sleep.
- *Stage 2: proper sleep.* This phase usually lasts about 30–40 minutes and although it doesn't take much to wake you up, you're likely to feel groggy.
- *Stages 3 and 4: deep sleep.* In stage 3, brainwaves give way to the slowest brainwaves – the delta waves. By stage 4, not much is going to wake you – a stampede of elephants could come charging through your room and you won't even stir, although amazingly hearing a familiar name could possibly rouse you. Your oxygen levels, heart rate and breathing levels are at their lowest. Now the

growth hormone is released, which helps cell renewal, building new tissue and repairing damaged cells.

■ *Stage 5: REM sleep*. This is when you have your most vivid dreams. Although you're not aware of it, your body and brain come to life – your brain is as active as it is when you're awake. Your eyes dart about, while your heart rate, breathing rate and blood pressure all rise and can be erratic – this explains those moments when you wake up from a disturbing dream with your heart thumping. Brainwaves speed up and slow down dramatically. Your memory is also being recharged. Most of us have gone to bed trying without success to remember something, only to find that when we awake the next morning the answer pops into our head as if by magic. Apart from finger and facial twitching, most of your muscles become paralysed to stop you acting out your dreams.

These stages alternate throughout the night and most people normally wake up for a few seconds, five times an hour – although they won't remember it. The exact pattern varies from person to person and with age. Babies spend about half their sleeping time in REM sleep, adults about a quarter. If you miss out on sleep, it's the lighter stages of sleep – 1 and 2 – that tend to be lost. The body will always do its best to catch up on deep sleep first, then REM sleep.

Find out how you can use your dreams to beat stress and sort out your problems in IDEA 28, *Dreamworks*.

Try another idea…

'Life is something you do when you can't get to sleep.'
FRAN LEBOWITZ, US writer

Defining idea…

3

How did it go?

Q **As soon as the traffic starts outside the house at 5.30 in the morning I wake up. Why am I woken so easily?**

A *During the early part of the night you spend more time in non-REM sleep and less time in REM sleep. As the night progresses, sleep is lighter, you wake up more and spend more time in REM sleep. By early morning almost all your sleep is REM sleep – which is why you can often remember your dreams at this time rather than the middle of the night.*

Q **If muscles are paralysed during sleep, why does my husband wake up with an erection every morning?**

A *No one really knows. Men get erections and women's vaginas become engorged every single time a person dreams, as often as three to five times a night. However, your husband is just as likely to be dreaming about diesel trains as what his secretary looks like with no clothes on. Sexual thoughts or dreams are not thought to trigger these responses.*

Q **You didn't mention why we sleep. Is there an explanation?**

A *Science still cannot explain why we sleep – in fact, most of the reasons given for sleep such as repairing tissues and conserving energy could be met by simply resting rather than going into an unconscious state. That said, it's worth finding out about what happens when we sleep – one study found that knowing the basics about sleep patterns reduced insomnia by 50%.*

The rhythms of life

Understand your body clock – and determine all your energy highs and lows in the day.

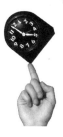

Brainwaves shape your sleep, but it's your body clock that tells you when it's time to go to bed in the first place.

Unlike the ticking clock swallowed by the crocodile in Peter Pan, however, you're unlikely to hear it. If you could, though, you'd hear a gushing release of hormones, your pumping heart and bubbling blood pressure – all timed to get you in the right state for going to sleep or waking up.

Your body clock normally works to a daily 24-hour cycle – and controls the release of hormones, blood pressure and heart rate plus when your body wants to go to sleep and wake up. We're programmed to fall asleep at night, when it's dark and cooler, and to be awake when it's light and warmer. Your body clock controls your temperature and sleepiness so that at night your temperature drops as you go to sleep and rises as you wake.

It also makes sure you don't have inconvenient appetites or needs – like going to the toilet or feeling hungry. An overwhelming desire to eat a cheese sandwich at 3 in the morning is certainly going to be disruptive on a regular basis.

Here's an idea for you...

Your body clock controls your movements in the day too – over 24 hours, you get restless and need a change of pace every 90 to 120 minutes. Observe these changes one day – see how you get up from your desk, stretch, have a cup of coffee, then get back to work, stop for lunch, have a cup of tea and so on. This broken regimen continues through the night as you change sleep stages.

You have another drop in temperature and sleepiness around midday until two in the afternoon. So when you feel like falling asleep on your computer at work, it's not necessarily because you stayed up all night watching horror videos – it's just your body clock telling you that a snooze would be nice, thank you. And the siesta is not just a product of a lazy Mediterranean lifestyle – it's encouraged by the controls in your brain.

PERFECT TIMING

The really clever thing is how the body knows what time it is. The key, it seems, is light. In the morning light enters the eye and hits the retina. This travels along nerves and ends up in a part of your brain responsible for regulating your body clock called the suprachiastmatic nucleus (SCN). Here signals are sent to the pineal gland in your brain to stop producing melatonin, the brain's sleep-inducing

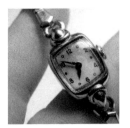

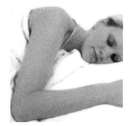

hormone and to release the get-up-and-go hormone cortisol. In the evening at around 10p.m. the fading light of the setting sun triggers melatonin to prepare your body for sleep. Once you're asleep, if you suddenly put on a light – to go to the toilet, for instance – chances are you'll have trouble dropping off again. This is because light kickstarts those get-up-and-go hormones, and as far as they're concerned it's wake-up time.

To find out if your body clock's running too fast or too slow, take a look at IDEA 3, *Lark or owl?*

Try another idea…

The average body clock is happiest when you sleep from around 11p.m. to 7a.m., which is when all the hormones are programmed to be either released or stopped. That said, everyone's body clock is set slightly differently and some run slower or faster than the average.

By studying these clocks, scientists are beginning to understand jet lag, and sleep problems such as insomnia and how to treat them. They are looking at the chemicals that govern sleep and making synthetic versions for supplements that in future may be able to help millions of people with sleep disorders. Some studies suggest that the hormone melatonin, given as a supplement at specific times, may be useful for resetting daily rhythms to help overcome the effects of jet lag and sleep disorders.

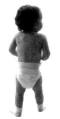

'Sleeping is no mean art: for its sake one must stay awake all day.'

FRIEDRICH NIETZSCHE

Defining idea…

How did
it go?

Q **I seem to want to sleep a lot more in winter. Do our body clocks change with the season?**

A *Darkness triggers your body clock to release sleep-inducing chemicals so in autumn, as it starts to get darker earlier, your body prepares for sleep earlier. The sun rises later, too, so your wake-up hormones are triggered later. This is why you sleep more in winter – and that getting out of bed seems as inviting as jumping naked off a cliff into ice cold water. According to the latest research, we need at least 30 minutes of sunlight a day to keep our body clocks in check so we want to fall asleep at the right time.*

Q **Can you reset a body clock?**

A *Yes, to a certain extent. You can fool your body that it's time to wake up with artifical light. Scientists have found that shining a bright light on the backs of our knees (of all places!) can reset the brain's sleep-wake clock. And British Ministry of Defence researchers have worked out how to reset soldiers' body clocks so they can go without sleep for up to 36 hours. Tiny optical fibres embedded in special glasses project a ring of bright white light (mimicking a sunrise) around the edge of soldiers' retinas, tricking them into thinking they've just woken up. The system was first used on US pilots during the bombing of Kosovo.*

Q **Are body clocks genetic?**

A *By studying mould, flies, mice and other organisms, scientists have learned that the function of the biological clock is controlled by specific genes. Obviously, this means the genes can be passed on. So if your parents are larks, chances are you'll be one too.*

3

Lark or owl?

Your eyelids start drooping after the early evening news or you're doing the mamba at midnight. Find out which one you are.

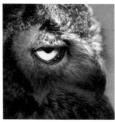

Do you have an overwhelming desire to iron a shirt at midnight, or maybe 5 in the morning would be your ideal time to go to the supermarket? Some 10% of us are up-at-dawn raring-to-go larks. About 20% are owls, and come to life in the evening.

Although most of us just bumble along, coping pretty well with the occasional late night or very early morning, some people's body clocks are slightly out of sync. Owls want to go to bed later and are slow to get going in the morning. They're normally seen running for a bus, still putting on their jackets, their stomachs groaning after missing breakfast. This is because their internal clocks run slightly slower than 24 hours and their daily cycle is longer. Owls often have trouble getting to sleep and stay in light sleep longer. If you find you want to do the laundry or surf the internet at midnight, you're probably an owl.

Here's an idea for you... **Write a list of which time in the day you are most alert and most productive. If you're a lark, it'll be some time between late morning and noon. If you're an owl, you'll get a short burst of productivity late morning, but you'll feel most alert around 6p.m. Then tailor your most challenging tasks around your up times.**

Larks' body clocks run slightly faster than 24 hours and their daily cycle is slightly shorter. So larks want to go to bed early, get up early and are irritatingly bright eyed and bushy tailed the minute they get up.

WORK TO YOUR CLOCK

Your body clock changes with time too. Generally we become more owl-like when we're teenagers and more lark-like when we get older. Whatever you are, there's not much you can do to change it. You just have to work around it – and that may mean finding a job that fits with your body clock. If you're a lark, you're going to be a hopeless bartender. If you're an owl, don't take that job presenting the morning news. You probably consider your lark/owl traits already when choosing a job – even if you're not aware of it. According to one study, casualty doctors are more likely to be owls than larks – as they spend more time working at night than any other doctors, this is very handy.

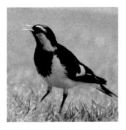

Although you can't change your basic make-up, there are tricks to help you adapt.

■ Workwise, it's easier if you're a lark as you'll have no trouble waking up – you might find after-work activities and socialising may suffer. If you want to stay up for a party, however, spend time out-side in the afternoon or early evening. Then go for a brisk walk or do some light stretching. This should help you stay up later and may help you sleep later in the morning. Sleep with curtains closed and, if you want to stay up later more regularly, consider buying black-out curtains which block out the light. Darkness tells you brain it's night-time – time to sleep.

■ If you're an owl and want to be more alert in the morning, keep your evenings quiet to help prepare your body for bed, sleep with curtains open and let daylight wake you up naturally. Walk outside as soon as possible after waking up. You should also do as much as you can the night before – select the next day's clothes for instance, so you don't have to think too hard in the morning.

If you're a night owl and find it difficult to go to bed any earlier, make sure your bedroom environment is conducive to sleep. Turn it into a sleep sanctuary in IDEA 38, *Snoozy rooms*.

Try another idea…

'Early to rise, and early to bed, makes a man healthy, wealthy and dead.'
Author, JAMES THURBER

Defining idea…

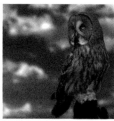

How did it go?

Q   I just can't get out of bed in the morning and I've tried all the tips you mentioned. Is there anything more extreme you can do to change my body clock?

A   *One method is so extreme you'll only be able to do it on holiday. This is to go to bed two hours later every couple of days until you work your way around the clock. So if you feel like going to bed at 2a.m. on the first day, you should go to bed at 4a.m., then the following two days at 6a.m. and so on. Once you've worked around the clock, you should stop at the time you want – then go to bed at this time every night. The only problem with this is that if you have one late night, it can take you back to where you were.*

Q   I'm a night owl and my girlfriend's a lark. We never seem to go to bed at the same time. What can we do?

A   *Conflict often occurs in couples where one is an early bird and the other a night owl. One is ready for sleep while the other is ready to rock and roll. Accept that you're not going to change, it's just part of who you are. Then you can negotiate a few nights a week when you go to bed at the same time. In truth, night owls would probably be happier in relationships with other night owls.*

Q   I'm always half asleep when I get to work. I can't function properly until about 11a.m. How can I be more productive in the morning?

A   *First, be honest with your colleagues. Apologise for seeming slower in the morning, and blame your body clock owl tendencies. You might be the butt of a few twit twoo jokes, but if your colleagues can help you work around your body clock then it's worth it. They can help you schedule more difficult tasks and meetings for the afternoon when you're more alert. If there's an option for flexible working hours, you should consider taking it.*

4

System failure

**Injury, poor performance and depression – the results of
not getting your sleep quota.**

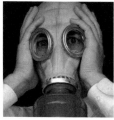

You're tired during the day, you're irritable,
anxious, have difficulty concentrating and
are about as alert as a fridge freezer.
If you don't deal with your sleep problem, your
health will spiral downwards and your once cheery
personality will be replaced by a glum, short-
tempered one. Here's what to expect ...

You probably don't need a scientist to tell you how rotten you're feeling after a
few bad nights. But it may be useful to know what's happening to your body when
you're deprived of sleep. It could be worse than you think ...

Here's an idea for you... **Set yourself a test to find out how lack of sleep affects you. Write down the names of 10 random objects which you then need to recall on another piece of paper. Time yourself when you do the test feeling rested, and compare the results after doing it again when you're sleep deprived. Obviously, change the test when you do it the second time.**

■ *Poor memory.* During a good night's sleep, in the REM stage, the brain busily replenishes the neurotransmitters that organise neural networks vital for remembering, learning, performance and problem solving. If you deprive the brain of sleep, you get less REM sleep. The result? The crossword takes twice as long to finish, you'll forget the names of close friends and you'll stare at the tax form for days before even attempting to fill it out.

■ *More car accidents.* According to one study drowsiness or sleep disorders was a factor in about half of all traffic accidents and 36% of fatal accidents. Another study compared the reaction times between people who were sleep deprived and those who'd been drinking alcohol. The result? Pretty poor mental functioning all round. This suggests that driving when tired is as dangerous as driving drunk

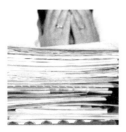

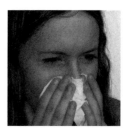

- *Constant colds.* With a tissue pressed to your face at all times, no one's really seen you properly for weeks – which is probably a good thing considering your dry, flaky red nose, cracked lips and streaming eyes. Recent research demonstrated that the nightly loss of four hours of sleep over 10 days in healthy young adults significantly reduced their immune function. This is because it reduces the number of white blood cells (which are responsible for the production of antibodies that fight disease).
- *Old before your time.* Research suggests that missing sleep can actually speed up ageing. Sleeping for only four hours a night for less than a week reduces the body's ability to process and store carbohydrates and regulate hormone levels

Worried about falling asleep at the wheel? Take a look at IDEA 20, *Dozy driving* and find out how to cope with driving when you're sleep deprived.

Try another idea...

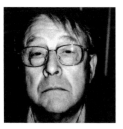

'Without enough sleep, we all become tall two-year-olds.'
JOJO JENSEN,
author of *Dirt Farmer Wisdom*

Defining idea...

– changes which are similar to those of advanced ageing. Another study found that sleeping under five hours per night shortened the life span (although sleeping more than nine hours also did the same).

- *Makes you fat.* Lack of sleep makes you hungry and more prone to putting on weight – one of the main causes of snoring and sleep apnoea. The key to this is the hormone leptin, which signals when the body needs or does not need more food. Leptin levels rise during sleep and this tells your brain that you've eaten enough and don't need any more calories. When you're sleep deprived, leptin levels are low, which sends a signal to your brain that you need more calories. Your brain thinks that there's a shortage of food and that you need to eat more, when in fact you've eaten enough.

- *High blood pressure.* Blood pressure usually falls during the sleep cycle; however, interrupted sleep can adversely affect this normal decline, leading to hyper-tension and cardiovascular problems. One study of nurses showed that those sleeping for five hours or fewer had a 45% greater risk of developing heart dis-ease than those sleeping for eight hours. Oversleeping also has risks, however. Those sleeping nine to eleven hours increased their risk by 38%.

- *Diabetes risk.* Research has also shown that insufficient sleep impairs the body's ability to use insulin, which can lead to the onset of diabetes.

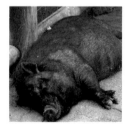

Q Can you die from insomnia?

How did it go?

A   *No you can't die from insomnia (although sometimes it may feel like it). It is not a disease, but a symptom.*

Q I'm an advertising creative and have to be on the ball at all times. Sometimes when I'm meeting a deadline I work through the night and I can barely speak the next day. Why is this?

A   *Your brain's frontal lobe, which is associated with speech as well as novel and creative thinking, is affected when you're deprived of sleep. So you might have trouble thinking of imaginative words or ideas – you're more likely to use repetitive words or clichéd phrases. Also, you might find it harder than normal giving a presentation – slurred speech, stuttering, speaking in a monotone voice, or speaking at a slower pace than usual are all signs of sleep deprivation. Studies show that sleep deprived people do not have the speed or creative abilities to cope with making quick but logical decisions. So although you'll understand a problem, you may well pick an unoriginal solution. The good news is, once you're sleeping normally again, you'll be as quick thinking and creative as you ever were.*

Q Do all your mental abilities deteriorate when you're sleep deprived?

A   *No. Research has suggested that basic arithmetic and maths isn't really affected by lack of sleep and, in some cases, even gets better.*

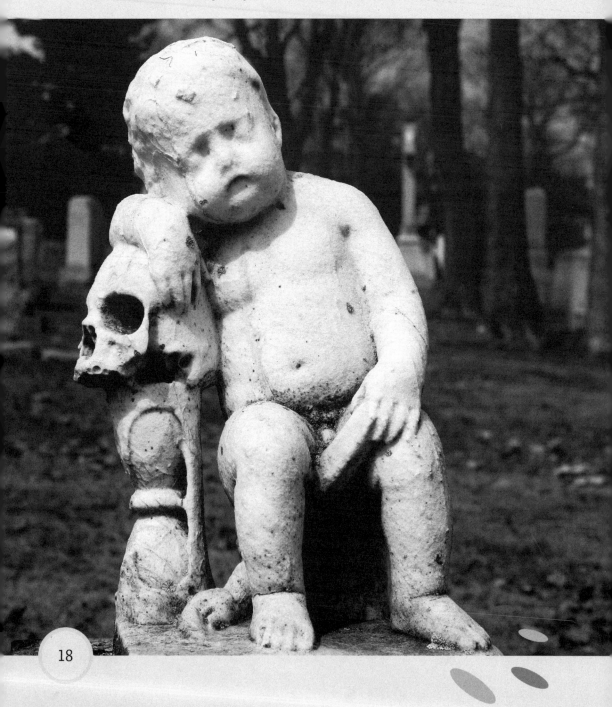

5

Six, seven or eight?

Margaret Thatcher survived on four hours, Napoleon six and Thomas Edison hardly slept at all, except in 20-minute naps. Are you getting enough to keep you on top form?

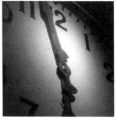

The average night's sleep now is about seven and a half hours — 90 minutes less than it was the 1920s. Ask anyone how much they think they should be getting and most people will say eight hours. But this ain't necessarily so.

Sleep experts don't normally talk in terms of number of hours, but the amount of sleep you need to be wide awake and alert in the day. So if you regularly fall asleep watching TV or reading or fall asleep in the car, you might not be getting enough.

That said, women seem to need about 20 minutes sleep more than men. The experts say it's because women use their brains in a more flexible way than men – which means their brains are working harder in the day and are therefore more tired at night.

Here's an idea for you…

To find out how many hours of sleep you need, carry out this test. For the next two weeks, record the amount of sleep you had during the night and rate your daytime functioning at the end of the day on a scale from 1(unable to think straight, constantly tired) to 10 (perfect performance). Rate how you performed at work, in your hobbies, in social situations and so on. After two weeks, look at the results and work out if your sleep has a direct link with how you function the next day. You might find that sleep length is not all that matters – six hours of uninterrupted sleep will be more refreshing than 9 hours of disturbed sleep.

Age plays a part too – in general the amount of sleep needed decreases with age. A baby can sleep up to 18 hours a day, a toddler 12–14, including a nap. By the time you're 60 you'll probably only need 5 or 6 hours a night. The amount of slow wave sleep, which is when the human growth hormone is secreted, is much higher in children and decreases with age. This is probably a good thing or we could all be the size of houses at the age of 50.

Remember being a teenager? Being told off for not going to bed, then being dragged out of bed in the morning half-asleep? Research now proves it wasn't your fault. A teenager's body clock actually resets so instead of producing the sleep-inducing melatonin earlier in the evening – like kids and adults – their body's not triggering it until 1 in the morning. So the average teenager would be much happier waking up at around 10. Until schools start their day at lunchtime, this isn't going to happen. In the meantime, teenagers who fall asleep after midnight may be missing out on one or two hours of sleep a night and find it hard to stay awake in class.

If you want to increase the amount of time you're asleep, don't suddenly go to bed an hour earlier than usual – you'll just lie awake in bed. Just go to bed 10 to 15 minutes earlier than usual every night until you're waking up refreshed. Then stick to this bedtime as much as possible so your body knows when to prepare for sleep.

Want to know what happens to you if you don't get enough sleep? Take a look at IDEA 4, *System failure* – guaranteed to scare you into bed by 10p.m. tonight, at the latest.

Try another idea…

There are cases when cutting back on sleep is good. For instance, the amount of sleep you need may actually drop if you are trying to cure insomnia. If you're lying awake for ages on your pillow unable to get to sleep, going to bed 15 minutes earlier is not going to do you any good. Generally sleep specialists say that you should be spending about 85% of your time in bed asleep. Sometimes cutting back on sleep for one night lifts the mood in depression people, but after going back to normal sleep, the depression normally returns.

If you're tired in the day, but your sleep schedule shows that you're getting enough sleep you could have a condition called tired all the time (TATT) which is characterised by low energy levels and needs to be treated with lifestyle changes such as doing more exercise and eating more healthily. However, it might be worth seeing your doctor in case of any underlying medical cause.

'A satisfying sleep, like a satisfying meal, can leave one happy and content, without feeling too full, and with room, perhaps, for just a little more.'

Sleep expert, JIM HORNE

Defining idea…

21

How did it go?

Q Can you really catch up on sleep?

A *Many people lose out on sleep during the working week, having less than six hours a night; they then make up for it at weekends. However, only about a third of this lost sleep needs to be regained, and it does not have to be recovered hour for hour. Much of the weekend sleep-in is not necessarily for recovery, but for enjoyment; even those people who have enough sleep during the week will indulge in a Sunday morning lie-in.*

Q Is too much sleep bad for you?

A *Yes – sleeping too much is a no-no. In one study people who admitted to spending 12 hours or more in bed were one and a half times more likely to die younger than those people who had less than nine hours shut-eye. Supporters of the theory that we are chronically deprived of sleep claim that several nights of nine-hour sleeps will make us feel better, but there is little evidence of this – in fact people who extend their sleep for many nights often take longer to fall asleep and find getting up in the morning no easier. Sleeping for long periods is also a sign of stress, depression and boredom.*

6

The big one

You struggle to keep your eyes open during the day, but can't get to sleep later on. Chances are, you've got insomnia ...

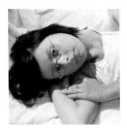

Nearly half of us suffer from insomnia every year, and frequently lie awake staring at the ceiling, unable to silence our babbling thoughts.

Insomnia is when you're not getting enough uninterrupted sleep to leave you refreshed the next day. Don't bother counting the minutes you were asleep. For a start, if you've got insomnia it's difficult to work out how long you've slept – it may well be more than you think. Also, because everyone needs a different amount of sleep, specialists don't think it's important – they're more interested in how poor sleep affects your ability to function in the day. For some people, a small loss of sleep can leave them unbelievably tired and irritable, totally unable to concentrate, taking them twice as long to carry out basic tasks.

The reason we have trouble sleeping varies from the mildly irritating – a cat whining outside your window – to whirring thoughts about work, financial difficulties

Here's an idea for you... **Work out what type of insomnia you have. Keep a sleep diary for three weeks. Write down how long it takes to get to sleep, how many times you wake up during the night and what time you wake up in the morning – plus how you felt the next day. After a few weeks you should see a pattern emerging. Now you can start to find solutions.**

or concern over a friend's illness. Sometimes it's just a free-floating anxiety that scoops up seemingly small worries like what colour to paint the bathroom or whether you were short-changed in the supermarket. It may be caused by medical illness, depression or a sleep disorder such as sleep apnoea.

Some 75% of insomnia will only last for a few nights and is caused by some change to your sleep schedule such as jet lag or illness. You may also be worried about a forthcoming event – a job interview perhaps – but once this has gone, your sleep will go back to normal. Women often suffer disturbed sleep during a period – body temperature rises causing tossing and turning. Short-term insomnia will last three to four weeks and is normally caused by events such as job loss, separation, divorce or health worries – if these are not dealt with it could lead to chronic insomnia. This is when your insomnia lasts over a month – and you get it regularly, or even every night.

WHICH TYPE ARE YOU?

Can't get to sleep? Normal sleepers take less than 20 minutes to fall asleep – if you're this type of insomniac it could take more than 30 minutes. In fact the average is just over an hour. You may find it difficult to get to sleep however tired you are. This is often due to anxiety, but it could be that your body clock is running too late.

Keep waking up in the night? Everyone wakes up momentarily throughout the night, but we're not aware of it so it doesn't affect our sleep. If you suffer this kind of insomnia, however, you wake up in the middle of the night, and spend what seems like ages, tossing and turning. You can be awake for hours or just wake up frequently. Triggers include snoring, sleep apnoea or sometimes depression.

Early morning insomnia? If you're an early bird or if you're used to waking up early for your job or your children, then getting up at the crack of dawn probably won't be a problem – particularly if you've gone to bed earlier to make up the time. If you've got early morning insomnia, however, you'll wake up more than an hour before you want to. Depression or a body that's set to wake up too early are common causes.

Defining idea...

'*Perhaps that's why some of us are insomniacs; night is so precious that it would be pusillanimous to sleep all through it!*'

Sci-fi author, BRIAN W ALDISS

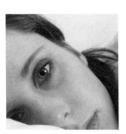

Try another idea...

To knock your sleep regime into shape, go to IDEA 7, *Back to basics*. You need to be tough, you need to be disciplined, but it'll be worth it in the end.

How did it go?

Q   When should I go to my doctor?

A   *When sleep is significantly ruining your daytime performance and continues for more than three weeks. Your doctor will investigate your insomnia – and if he or she suspects there's a medical cause such as sleep apnoea may refer you to a sleep clinic. If it's related to stress or depression, you may be referred to a counsellor. Insomnia is a symptom that something else is wrong, so if you tackle the cause, you're more likely to beat the insomnia.*

Q   Who's most likely to suffer?

A   *Insomnia is more common in older people and women are twice as likely to suffer than men. People with children are more likely to suffer although less than 3% of children report any serious problem of insomnia. Teenagers are famously sleep deprived – but that's normally a matter of choice. After the age of 50, insomnia gets more common and 45% of people over 80 complain of poor sleep on three or more nights a week.*

Q   Why do I always have trouble sleeping before I go on a trip abroad? I travel a lot through business – and I'm not even aware of being nervous about travelling. Once I've come back from my trip I'm fine.

A   *This is because you are associating travelling with a bad night's sleep. When you first started travelling, you probably were nervous and it affected your night's sleep. Now the thought of the next trip brings on a bout of insomnia, not because you're worried about travelling, but because you expect to have a bad night's sleep before the journey. Instead of thinking 'Oh, no, I'll get no sleep again,' say to yourself, 'I'm not nervous about travelling, I've done it lots of times before, and as long as I get some sleep, I'm sure I'll feel fine the next day.' This takes the pressure off a bit.*

7

Back to basics

Your journey to the land of sleep starts here – your first steps in beating insomnia.

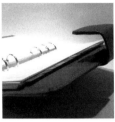

I'll start by helping you knock your sleep regime into shape. Just a warning, however. If your sleep pattern is as erratic as that of most insomniacs, this programme will be as enjoyable as a stay in a military boot camp.

- *Get a routine.* Go to bed and get up at the same time each day – no matter how bad your sleep has been. Your body clock needs a starting point, which is why the time you get up is so important. Also it's much easier to control when you get up – try to stay within 30 minutes of the same rising time every day.
- *Restrict your sleep.* This may sound odd advice for someone who is already sleep deprived, but spending too much time in bed can make insomnia worse. There's no point being in bed if you're not asleep – you'll just start associating bed with being awake. If you don't go to bed until you're really tired and get up early, the theory is you'll drop off more quickly, have less interrupted sleep and

Here's an idea for you... **To work out your sleep efficiency – the amount of time in bed actually asleep – you divide the time spent asleep by the time spent in bed and multiply this by one hundred. If you slept for 6 hours but were in bed for 9, your sleep efficiency is 66%.**

more deep sleep. Sleep scientists talk about sleep efficiency, which is the percentage of time you spend in bed asleep. A good sleeper will have a high sleep efficiency – around 90%. If you have 70% or less, think about reducing the time you spend in bed so that it more closely matches the time you're asleep.

– To decide when to go to bed, you need to work out how much sleep on average you're getting a night. The best way to do this is to use a sleep diary for a week. Once you've got a figure, add one hour. This should be the most time you spend in bed – and shouldn't be under five and a half hours – the average basic sleep requirement. So if you need to get up at 7a.m. and you need to sleep six hours, you shouldn't go to bed before 1a.m., no matter how tired you are.

– Once your sleep efficiency has improved to about 85% for two weeks, you can increase your time in bed by 15 minutes a week by going to bed 15 minutes earlier. Still get up at the same time, though. You may find that eight hours sleep a night is not necessary. Perhaps six or seven hours of better sleep are enough to feel good and function well during the day.

- *Get out of bed in the night.* Instead of lying awake, you could get up, go into another room and so something relaxing like listening to relaxing music, reading or relaxation exercises. When your eyelids start to droop, then return to your bed. Again, the idea is to associate bed with sleep.

'If you can't sleep, then get up and do something instead of lying there worrying. It's the worry that gets you, not the lack of sleep.'

DALE CARNEGIE, self-help guru

Defining idea...

- *Use bright light therapy.* Exposure to light boxes (similar to those used by seasonal affective disorder or SAD sufferers) helps people whose body clocks are out of sync. The idea is that bright light in the evening slows down the body clock while bright light in the morning speeds it up. If you can't get to sleep and find it difficult to stay asleep or you're a night owl who can't go to bed until the early hours of the morning, your body clock is lagging behind normal. So sitting in front of bright light in the morning for at least an hour brings the body clock forward. If, however, you wake up too early, your body clock is running faster than normal. You need bright light in the evening to slow your body clock down – just 30 minutes can cure early morning insomnia in some people.

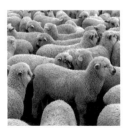

Think yourself sleepy with the fabulous mental tricks in IDEA 32, *Mind power* – you'll be amazed what your brain can do!

Try another idea...

How did it go?

Q   I fall asleep easily, but wake very early and can't get back to sleep. I've tried sleep restriction therapy but according to the theory I should be going to bed at midnight. But I can barely keep my eyes open after about 9.30. What should I do?

A   *Sounds like you have a lark body clock which makes it very difficult to stay up late. You'll have to juggle with the times a bit. If your ideal wake-up time is 7.30, and you need six hours sleep, push this back to 5.30 and try to stay up until 11.30. If this is too late, you may have to go slowly. Start going to bed at 10.30 and add 15 minutes every week or so until your body clock adjusts. Try to do stimulating activities like sewing, ironing, bill sorting, catching up with emails in the evening rather than passive ones like watching television.*

Q   I often wake up in the night unable to get back to sleep. I've tried getting out of bed, but this just wakes me up even more. What can I do?

A   *Fair enough, if it doesn't work for you. Try out things that might. Keep headphones by your bed. You could put on a relaxation tape or music that makes you drift off. Read in bed – but use a book light so it doesn't disturb your partner. Or learn a bunch of in-bed relaxation exercises that you can perform in the middle of the night.*

8

Wired!

Can't function without your morning coffee? Why stimulants can play havoc with your sleep cycle.

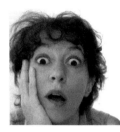

Why is it that the very things that help you stay alert are going to ruin your chances of a decent night's sleep? Life's just so unfair ...

CAFFEINE

Your morning coffee works for a reason. Caffeine stimulates the central nervous system (brain and spinal chord), increasing your metabolic rate, blood pressure, heart rate and breathing levels. It also blocks the effects of adenosine, a natural sedative found in the brain which builds up during the day and triggers the adrenal glands to produce the stimulating hormone adrenaline. It works fast, too. Caffeine, which is found in coffee, tea, cola and chocolate, is absorbed in only 15–30 minutes but its effects can last longer than four hours. No wonder caffeine makes it more difficult to get to sleep and reduces the quality of sleep. Studies show that having a caffeinated drink at night makes you wake up more often – it's particularly thought to reduce deep sleep and REM sleep.

Here's an idea for you...

If you want to drink less alcohol at home, use a tall, slim glass. Research has shown that we serve ourselves 20% more when using a short, wide glass than when the glass is tall and slim. Yet we assume we're drinking less from a short glass and more from a tall one.

That said, one of the best sleepers I know can take a double espresso ten minutes before sleep and have no trouble dropping off. It seems some people are better at metabolising caffeine, maybe because they're used to consuming more.

Cutting down

- Limit yourself to two cups of coffee or three or four of tea, but don't have them too late in the day.
- If you're relying on coffee to give you energy, go for snacks such as a banana, dried fruit or a cereal bar, which will do the trick just as well.
- Replace one of your daily teas or coffees with an alternative. Choose from herbal tea, milk shake, fruit juice, smoothie or even decaffeinated tea or coffee.

ALCOHOL

If you've had a few drinks, you're not likely to have much trouble getting to sleep – probably on the stairs on the way up to bed. But you'll probably wake up again as alcohol has just as disruptive an effect on sleep as caffeine. Although it's a sedative, it causes the release of adrenaline and blocks tryptophan, which helps the body make the calming brain chemical serotonin – vital for sleep. One unit of alcohol (half a pint of beer, one small glass of wine) takes about one hour to metabolise. So if you drink three glasses of wine at 10p.m., expect your sleep to be disrupted from around 1a.m. Again some people metabolise it faster than others.

Cutting down

- Have at least two drink-free days a week.
- Don't drink more than two units of alcohol per day if you're a women, three units if you're a man.
- Alternate an alcoholic drink with a non-alcoholic one such as non-alcoholic beer, water or a soft drink.
- Sip your drink slowly so it lasts longer.
- Try to eat before you go drinking since it will help reduce the amount of alcohol absorbed by your body.

'I always keep a stimulant handy in case I see a snake, which I also keep handy.'
WC FIELDS

Defining idea...

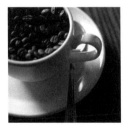

You now know what to avoid. Find out what you should be eating to ensure a good night's sleep in IDEA 33, *Food for thought*.

Try another idea...

NICOTINE

The increased risk of cancer and heart disease not a good enough reason to make you give up smoking? Well, this one might work. The average smoker takes twice as long to fall asleep as a non smoker and sleeps 30 minutes less. You may feel relaxed after having a cigarette, but it's probably because you've satisfied the craving rather than anything in nicotine. In fact, like caffeine it's a powerful stimulant and triggers the release of adrenaline. Like alcohol, once metabolised, nicotine can wake you up. Nicotine can cause difficulty falling asleep, problems waking in the morning, and may also cause nightmares.

Cutting down

There's no cutting down, you've got to bite the bullet and quit.

- If you're a woman, don't pack it in in the second half of your menstrual cycle, though. Researchers have found that you're much more likely to succeed if you do it in the first half because nicotine withdrawal symptoms – depression, anxiety and irritability – are worse in the second half.
- If you can use simply willpower, that's great. Otherwise there's a host of options from nicotine patches and self-help manuals to acupuncture and hypnotherapy. None of these will work unless you really want to give up, though.

Q **I've cut out coffee completely. Why have I got a headache?**

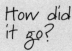

How did it go?

A *Cutting out caffeine suddenly can cause symptoms such as headaches, restlessness and irritability. Caffeine, you see, acts as a powerful vasocon-strictor – it constricts blood vessels in the brain and decreases circulation! When caffeine is not present, the sudden increased circulation causes headaches. These will only last a few days. Cut out one cup of coffee or tea a day over the course of several days and you'll probably avoid them.*

Q **Chocolate's my greatest pleasure. Do I have to give it up to get a good night's sleep?**

A *Don't worry, you won't have to give up your chocolate treats. You'd need to eat over ten 150g bars of dark chocolate, 30 bars of milk chocolate or 50 cups of hot chocolate to have any real effect. As a rule, the darker the chocolate, the more caffeine it contains.*

Q **Has all coffee got the same amount of caffeine?**

A *Real coffee has twice the caffeine content of instant coffee and strong tea is not far short of instant coffee.*

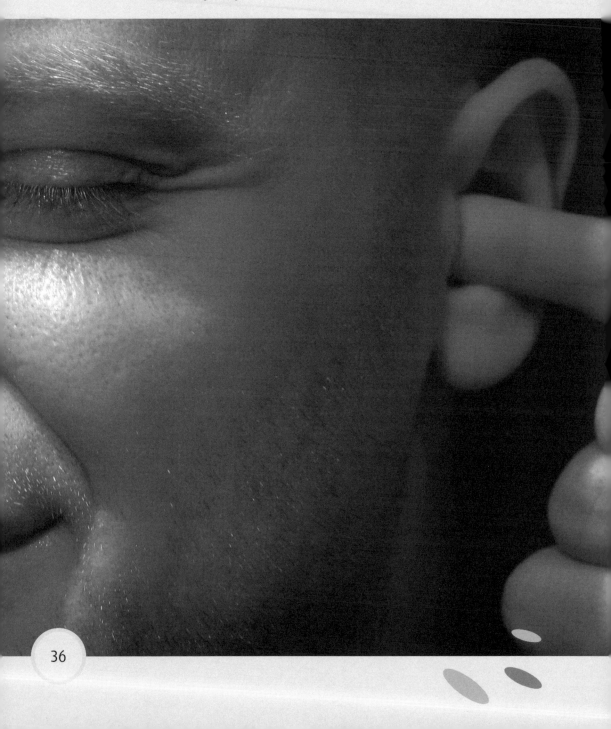

9

Noisy nights!

It sounds like a neighbour doing some late night drilling, but it is in fact your snoring bed partner. Act now before snoring ruins your sleep – and your relationship.

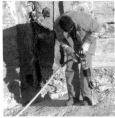

Although seen as a joke, and almost always denied by the snorer ('Well, I can't hear anything') snoring can be a serious issue between couples. Not surprising when you consider that loud snoring costs sleeping partners an average of one hour's sleep a night.

Snoring is the noise of tissues vibrating as air tries to flow through a blocked breathing passage. The sound can vary from an almost soothing whisper to an astonishingly loud noise that can be heard throughout the entire house.

Here's an idea for you...

If you meet a snorer at a party, ask them to do this test – guaranteed to break the ice. Ask them to stick their tongue out as far as it will go, grip it between their teeth, then try to make a snoring noise. If the snoring noise is reduced with their tongue in this forward position then they're probably a 'tongue base snorer'. This means their tongue is dropping to the back of their throat, causing a blockage. Tell your new friend they can buy small gum shields that gently bring their lower jaw forward or see their dentist about other jaw repositioning devices.

Don't waste time trying too many treatments, though – it's much more useful to find the cause of your snoring and tackle that. This checklist should help.

- *Are you overweight?* Find out by checking your Body Mass Index (BMI). You can do this by dividing your weight (kg) by your height squared (m). If your BMI is greater than 25 you are overweight. If your BMI is greater than 30 you are obese. Another measure is your collar size – over 16.5 inches and you're likely to snore because the muscles around your windpipe can't support the fat around it when you're asleep. In all these cases you need to lose weight – even a small loss can improve symptoms.
- *Do you smoke or drink?* Cigarette smoke irritates the lining of the nasal cavity and throat causing swelling and catarrh.

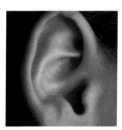

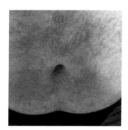

If the nasal passages become congested it's difficult to breathe through your nose because there's less airflow. And because congestion gets worse with each cigarette, the more you smoke, the worse your snoring. Even passive smoking can cause chronic inflammation of the nose and throat passages, thus increasing the risk of snoring. Until you give up don't smoke for at least 4 hours before bed.

Drinking triggers snoring as it reduces the tone of the muscles that keep the upper breathing passage open. So keep to the limit and avoid drinking just before bedtime.

- *Do you breathe through your mouth?* Open your mouth and make a snoring noise. Now close your mouth and try to make the same noise. If you can only snore with your mouth open then you are a 'mouth breather'. You'll probably wake up with a dry mouth and sometimes a sore throat because of the strain of snoring. When we breathe in through the nose the air passes over the curved part of the soft palate in a gentle flow into the throat without creating unnecessary turbulence. When we breathe in through the mouth, however, the air hits the back of the throat head on and can create

Is your snoring followed by silent periods, then a gasping for breath? If so, you could have sleep apnoea. Turn to IDEA 21, *Snores you can't ignore*.

Try another idea…

'I think a woman married to a snorer should be granted a divorce without any argument'

Defining idea…

HV MORTON,
travel writer (1892–1979)

enormous vibrations in the soft tissue. Try to breathe through your nose – and ask your pharmacist for gadgets (such as chin strips) that help keep your mouth closed. To help clear your nose, put a few drops of eucalyptus on your pillow-case.

■ *Are your nostrils too narrow?* Looking in a mirror, press the side of one nostril to close it. With your mouth closed, breathe in through your other nostril. If the nostril tends to collapse try propping it open with the clean end of a match-stick. If breathing is easier with the nostril propped open (try both sides), you may need something to open your nasal airways. Small or collapsing nostrils can prevent you from breathing through your nose. This encourages mouth breathing, and it's the air hitting the back of the throat that causes the snor-ing noise. Try nasal strips which you place on the outside of the nostrils to stop them collapsing.

■ *Do you sleep on your back?* This can cause snoring as it allows the flesh of your throat to relax and block airways. Also the fatty tissue around your neck can add pressure on the airway. Sleep on your side, if possible. A well known trick is sleeping with a tennis ball sewn into the back of your pyjama top.

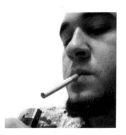

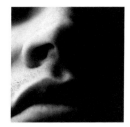

Q   Is snoring serious?

A   It's not normally a sign of a medical problem unless you've got sleep apnoea – so you won't be tired in the day, won't stop breathing at night and will have normal blood pressure. A doctor may check blood pressure or, if your nose is stuffy at night, may point to an allergy to a feather pillow or cat. Snoring can be caused by a broken nose, enlarged tonsils or a jaw that is set too far back but if there's no medical problem, your doctor won't recommend surgery.

Q   My wife and I are both overweight. How come I snore and she doesn't?

A   Men tend to put on weight around their necks and waists, whereas women seem to put on weight around the thighs. So when you lay on your back your fatty tissue adds pressure onto the airway, blocking it off and making you snore. Your wife's airway is not collapsing – not just because of where her weight is, but because women's airway walls tend to be less flexible and therefore less prone to yield to pressure when they're asleep.

Q   I always go to bed before my partner because of his snoring, but I feel we're missing out on bedtime intimacy. What can we do?

A   If the snoring cures I mention don't work, it's worth considering separate bedrooms if you have the space. Just get together for sex and go into your separate rooms to sleep.

How did it go?

41

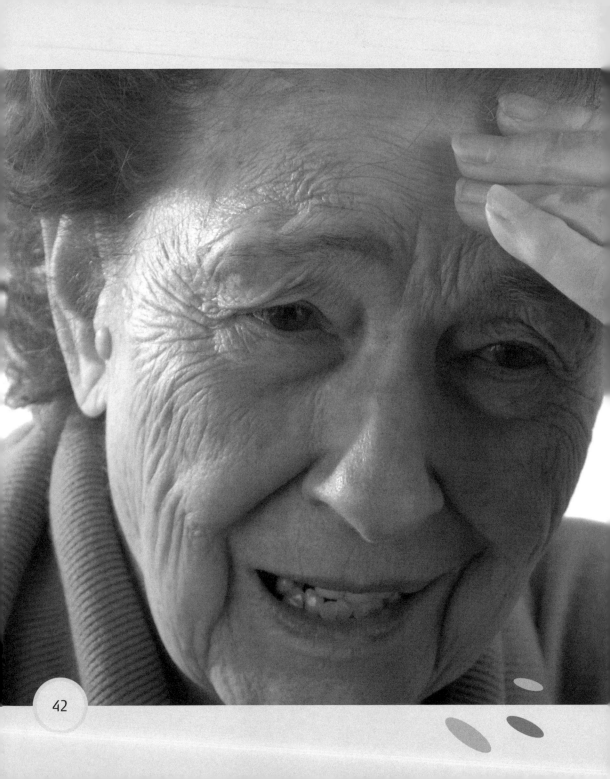

10

All stressed out!

Juggling work and home life? Busier than ever? You're probably stressed – it's the number one cause of insomnia.

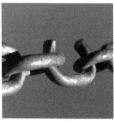

Your boss is putting pressure on you to stay late at work, you're not seeing enough of your kids, you still keep getting those headaches, you haven't agreed what colour to paint the hall and the man still hasn't come to repair your washing machine. It's no wonder you can't sleep and your relationship is suffering.

Today's lifestyles are busier than they've ever been. We work longer hours than ever before – and survey after survey says many of us are worn out and disillusioned with our jobs. Three in every five workers now complain of being stressed at work, the main cause being increased workloads, change at work, staff cuts, long hours and bullying. And some 84% of women say they're expected to perform too many roles and 74% think that overwork is damaging their health.

Here's an idea for you...

Start a stress diary. For at least two weeks, keep a list of events, times, places and people that seem to make you feel more stressed. You'll probably be surprised to find that a pattern soon emerges. For instance, you may be sensitive to time pressure – an approaching deadline or the daily grind of getting the kids dressed and ready by 8 o'clock for the school run. Perhaps personality clashes with certain people at work cause a sudden rise in stress levels. Or you could worry about social events like parties and all that small talk. Maybe people making inappropriate demands causes your anxiety. Or it could be a case of you simply trying to do too many things at once. Once you've identified your pressure points you can work out how to deal with them.

With expectations skyrocketing all the time – we now want the perfect relationship, a beautiful home, model children, a high performance car and wonderful holidays – it's no surprise that stress levels are at an all-time high as we fail to meet these unachievable goals. It only needs a stressful life event such as a divorce or death, moving home or a new job to tip you over the edge.

A certain amount of stress is good for us – it makes us perform better. In the past a shot of adrenaline and cortisol would pump us up for fighting enemies or running away from danger. The problem today is that instead of just using these stress hormones in emergencies, we are now living at such a pace that we activate them all the time – like when we're going to miss a train, or when someone records over our favourite video tape. The result? Sleep problems …

Stress not only makes it more difficult to sleep because the stress hormones are keeping your mind active, but it also depletes the sleep hormones serotonin and melatonin so you can't relax. On top of this, stress reduces the amount of deep sleep you get, making the sleep you do get lighter and less satisfactory. And you're more likely to wake up in the middle of the night. Then, of course, you get anxiety dreams – who hasn't suffered the humiliation of walking through their office with no clothes on? Fortunately, however, for most people, sleep returns to normal when the factor causing the stress is removed.

Finished your stress diary? Check out IDEA 22, *Say no to stress*, to find out how to take control of your stress triggers.

Try another idea…

If you're wondering which gender is more affected, it seems women are better at coping with stress. Some say it's because some female hormones seem to protect them from the effects of stress – others say they're simply better at talking about the causes of their stress, which is one of the keys to stopping it. And middle aged men may be more prone to insomnia caused by stress because it seems they're more vulnerable to stress hormones. As men age they seem to become more sensitive to the stimulating effects of cortisol when they're trying to go to sleep.

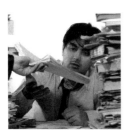

'A ruffled mind makes a restless pillow.'
CHARLOTTE BRONTE

Defining idea…

45

Q   Sometimes news events get me down. Can the news cause stress?

A   *Yes you can get stressed by things that are beyond your control and related to factors that are completely outside your environment. After the September 11 attack there was a huge increase in cases of insomnia in the US even though most were nowhere near New York and knew no one who'd been killed. It's thought many people were suffering from post-traumatic stress disorder, a condition where people keep reliving a traumatic event in their head, making them withdrawn and depressed. Try not to watch or listen to the news in the evening or before you go to bed – you might find it hard to put the words and images out of your mind.*

Q   Why do some people lose sleep during periods of stress, while others seem to sleep like a baby?

A   *For a start, some people are just better sleepers and are less affected by stress. But the way you cope with stress has an affect too. One study found that people who fret and brood as a way to cope with stress were more likely to suffer sleep loss, while those who tended to ignore emotions and focus on tasks extended their sleep and shut themselves off from stress. The lesson? Don't wallow in your emotions, but do something constructive to sort your stress.*

11

Baby on the way

You've got swollen ankles, sore breasts and a tummy the size of a spacehopper, and to make matters worse you haven't had a decent night's sleep for weeks.

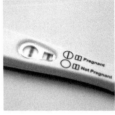

When you're staring at the ceiling at 3 in the morning, it might console you to know that you're not alone — some 80% of pregnant women complain of disturbed sleep.

As a rule, most symptoms get worse as your bump gets bigger. Oh the joys of pregnancy! Here's what to expect – then what to do about it.

0–3 MONTHS

Although most women's sleep remains normal, some women suffer poor sleep from the beginning. This is probably due to the effect on the brain of the rising levels of the hormone progesterone which – rather unfairly – not only makes you feel drowsy in the day, it can also disrupt your sleep at night, leading to even more fatigue during the next morning. Nausea could also keep you awake. The most

Here's an idea for you... **Still uncomfortable? Lie on your side with your knees bent and a pillow between your knees. Arrange other pillows under your belly and behind your back for extra support.**

common reason for disrupted sleep, however, is going to the toilet. When I was pregnant, I seriously considered camping out in the bathroom – with so many trips to the toilet, I worked out I'd have saved up to an hour of precious sleep time in one night.

3–6 MONTHS

You might find you're more tired, go to bed, but then are awake most of the time tossing and turning, trying to find a comfortable position. At its most extreme this turns into restless legs syndrome – unpleasant tingling sensations in the legs which lead to an uncontrollable urge to move. You may suffer cramps in your calves as your leg muscles struggle to cope with the extra weight.

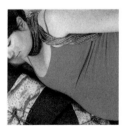

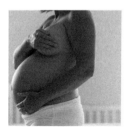

You could also start to get heartburn at night. This is caused by acid from the stomach going backward into the oesophagus, the tube that carries food from the throat to the stomach. This may be triggered by the growing uterus putting extra pressure on your stomach.

6–9 MONTHS

Irritated by your husband's snoring? Well it might be his turn to complain. You may develop nasal congestion, which could cause you to snore for the first time in your life. Also prepare for severe back pains that interfere with your sleep. Then there are the frightening dreams, which are more surreal than normal. I once dreamt about giving birth to a giant spider, a terrifying image I couldn't shake off for weeks. Towards the end of pregnancy, the discomfort and movement of your baby could mean you're awake nearly all night. And your baby isn't even born yet …

Got an irresistible urge to move your legs at night? Find out more about restless legs syndrome in IDEA 12, *Itches and twitches*

Try another idea…

'By far the most common craving of pregnant women is not to be pregnant.'
PHYLLIS DILLER, comedienne

Defining idea…

49

SLUMBER STRATEGIES

- Don't drink an hour or two before bed to limit night-time trips to the toilet.
- Since nausea tends to strike an empty stomach, eat a light, high-carbohydrate snack before you go to bed and keep some crackers or rice cakes on your night table so it's easy to grab one in the morning.
- If you get heartburn at night, avoid distending your stomach by eating small, frequent meals rather than three large ones. Lay off the citrus, spices, fried foods and chocolate because they can irritate the oesophagus. Sit up after eating. Sleeping on several pillows might help. If it persists, see your doctor who might prescribe an antacid.
- Train yourself to sleep on your side. Sleeping flat on the back can restrict breathing and may reduce blood flow to the baby if the uterus presses on the main artery of your body, the aorta.
- If you have restless legs syndrome (RLS), you may have been deficient in iron or folic advice before becoming pregnant – your doctor may prescribe vitamin supplements.
- To stop cramps, try stretching your calf by flexing your foot heel first, gently massaging your leg, placing a hot water bottle on the cramped area, or getting up and walking around.

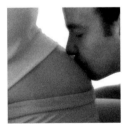

Q   **I wake in the middle of the night panicking that I'll be a bad parent, never be able to cope or simply forget where I put the baby. What can I do?**

How did it go?

A   *The only way to stop these perfectly natural fears is to get prepared: read books, and take a childbirth preparation class. Confide in your partner, too, who may be feeling the same way you are. Bringing your fears out into the open may help you deal with them.*

Q   **Will my lack of sleep harm my baby?**

A   *Relax – your baby can sleep even when you're wide awake. No one knows why your baby sleeps independently of you, though we do know that the need to sleep is one our strongest physiological drives. We also know that a baby isn't bothered by the same sounds that keep you awake: layers of skin and muscle, as well as amniotic fluid, insulate your baby from outside noise and movement. But your baby's not completely cut off from what's going on around him: a sharp noise or sudden movement can wake him up, and you may feel a kick or punch as a result.*

Q   **I've heard sleeping on the left side is better – is this true, and if so why?**

A   *Although there's no real harm in sleeping on your right side, lying on your left side is actually good for you and your baby: it improves the flow of blood and nutrients to the placenta and it helps your kidneys efficiently eliminate waste products and fluids from your body. That, in turn, reduces swelling in your ankles, feet and hands. If you train yourself to sleep on your left side early on, you'll have an easier time falling asleep when your belly is bulging later.*

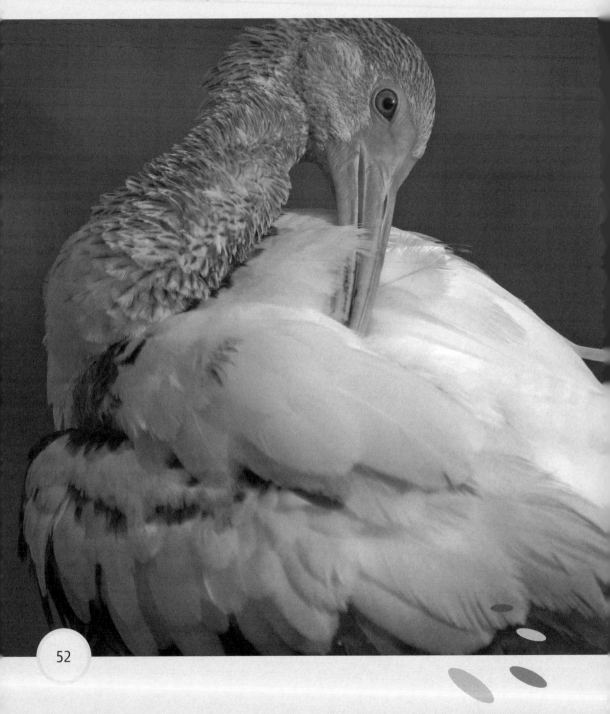

12

Itches and twitches

From tossing and turning to constant kicking, why some people can't stop moving all night long.

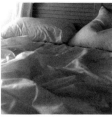

As soon as you lie down in your bed, you get a creepy crawly feeling in your legs making it impossible for you to find a comfortable position. Moving your legs is your only relief so you end up tossing and turning all night. If this sounds like you, you could have restless legs syndrome ...

The main symptom of restless legs syndrome (RLS) is an unpleasant burning, prickling, tickling or aching feeling in your leg muscles, mainly in the calf, when you're inactive or relaxing – which is why it's worse at night. You'll have an irresistible urge to move your legs which is only relieved by actually moving them. In the day, it just makes you fidget – at night you'll probably have to keep changing position or you might even have to get out of bed and walk around. Some people also suffer involuntary jerking movements in their legs – so don't be surprised if your bed part-

Here's an idea for you…

Track your progress. Keep a record of how any changes in lifestyle affect the symptoms of restless legs syndrome and the quality of your sleep. Every three days try something new so you can establish what makes a difference. Give each strategy a mark out of 10 where 1 is 'useless' and 10 is 'worked like a dream'.

ner wakes up black and blue, complaining of being kicked in the stomach all night. Chances are, you – and possibly your partner – are sleep deprived. You're probably taking more than half an hour to get to sleep and could be waking up three or more times in the night.

WHO GETS IT?

Up to 15% of people suffer – some only mildly, others finding it almost impossible to get an uninterrupted night's sleep. It tends to run in families, it's more common in women and the risk goes up as you get older. Pregnant women are also more prone.

WHAT CAUSES IT?

No one really knows this – no detectable abnormality of the nervous system, circulation or muscles has been found. However, RLS has been associated with other conditions, which if treated, can help. For instance, restless legs can be a symptom of a deficiency in iron, vitamin B12 or folic acid, and taking supplements will normally sort it out. Nerve damage associated with rheumatoid arthritis, kidney failure or diabetes may also cause RLS – but once the underlying condition is treated, RLS will probably get better. Certain medications including lithium, anticonvulsants, antidepressants and beta-blockers are also thought to be triggers – so changing to other drugs can help. Smoking, drinking alcohol and having too much caffeine seems to make RLS symptoms worse – so cut down or cut them out.

ACTION PLAN

- Stick to a regular sleep routine – irregular sleep habits may make you more tired and make RLS symptoms worse. So go to bed and wake up at the same time every day if possible. Work out how many hours you need to feel refreshed, and adjust your sleep schedule. If possible go to sleep later and wake up later. If you've got RLS, you're more likely to sleep better later in the night – from about 2a.m. to 10a.m.

- Test out different pre-bed rituals to see what works for you. Good ones to try are pacing up and down, performing a stretching routine that includes leg work, taking a hot or cold bath, massaging your legs with oil or applying hot or cold packs. Some people swear by TENs machines, which are often used during labour as a drug-free way of easing the pain of contractions: you put pads on your legs which are attached via wires to a stimulator. These emit vibrating electrical impulses which block the aching and tickling sensations in your leg. To distract you, read a novel or try a relaxation technique such as meditation or yoga.

- If lifestyle changes don't work, there are a huge amount of drugs, such as levodopa, bromocriptine, oxycodone and clonazepam, that are used to control RLS: they work in different ways by stopping the restlessness, abnormal sensations, involuntary movements, anxiety and by relaxing muscles. However, it's a complicated process – so your doctor will have to tailor-make a treatment programme for you.

Let the irritating sensation in your legs wash over you completely by learning how to meditate. Turn to IDEA 43, Ommmm …, for a pre-bed routine, or distract yourself with one of the mental tricks in IDEA 32, Mind power.

Try another idea…

'*In young people restless legs syndrome is misdiagnosed as growing pains.*'
Dr TRISHA MACNAIR

Defining idea…

Q   Should I exercise?

A   *Regular moderate exercise may help, but too much can make symptoms worse so you may have to give up your training for the marathon. You should also not exercise at least six hours before bedtime – although stretching and walking seems to help some people prepare for sleep.*

Q   Should I fight the urge to move my legs at night?

A   *No. If you attempt to suppress the urge to move, you may find that your symptoms only get worse. Get out of bed if you have to. Find an activity that takes your mind off of your legs and do some gentle stretching.*

Q   Can I take medication during pregnancy?

A   *Best to stick to the lifestyle changes – there's a danger that the drugs may interfere with the development of the foetus, particularly in the first three months of pregnancy. Symptoms often get worse as pregnancy progresses – by the last three months, however, you may be able to take some low-risk drugs such as opoids, as there's a much lower risk of harm to your baby.*

13
What a grind!

Fingernails scratching a blackboard, a pneumatic drill and a rat gnawing through timbers... these are just some of the noises that have been used to describe teeth grinding. No wonder it can disrupt your sleep.

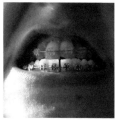

This habit, which can be as loud and disruptive as snoring, not only keeps your bed partner up half the night, it can mean you wake up with jaw ache or a splitting headache.

Teeth grinding – or bruxism if you want to get technical – is a condition where you either press, clench, or physically grind your teeth against each other. If you're one of the 10% of adults who suffer this at night, there's a chance you're doing it in the day, too, but you're not aware of it. Each episode of grinding lasts four to five seconds and happens about 25 times per night. If you or your partner are light sleepers, that's a lot of potential awakenings.

WHAT CAUSES IT?

No one really knows why people get it. It might simply be a habit like biting your nails, drumming fingers or sucking the inside of your cheeks – in fact, many teeth grinders also have these quirks. The most likely trigger, however, is stress. You may

Here's an idea for you... **Write down what sets off your teeth grinding in the day, then find an activity to do every time you feel the urge. This could be slow, deep breathing for instance. Or you could repeat a relaxing phrase – or even a favourite line of poetry – to distract you until the desire to grind passes. Place 'don't grind' reminders around the house on post-its. The idea is that if you break the habit during the day this may help stop the grinding at night.**

well be stressed if you're having difficulty concentrating, feeling more irritable than usual, you need a drink to relax or rely on comfort food. As a result you could be finding it difficult to get to sleep or having fitful sleep.

WHAT ARE THE SYMPTOMS?

You may wake up with a headache, jaw ache or earache that goes away as the day wears on. These are all are caused by joint and muscle strain in your upper and lower jaws. And if left untreated, the surface of your upper and lower teeth can be worn down so much it creates an imbalance in closure between the left and right sides of your mouth. This can lead to gum disease and you may even lose some of your teeth.

WHO SPOTS IT?

Normally your long suffering partner or your dentist who should detect the characteristic wear on the teeth. Wear associated with grinding is most evident on the molars in the back of your mouth. Have a look yourself by opening your mouth and checking your teeth in the mirror. You're a teeth grinder if your teeth are worn down on one side of your mouth or if the enamel that covers your teeth has worn down to reveal the slightly darker dentine beneath it.

To find out how to use a stress diary and other ways to cut your stress, check out IDEA 22, *Say no to stress*.

Try another idea…

HOW'S IT TREATED?

You need to tackle the cause – that means reducing stress – as well as stop the situation getting any worse – that means proper tooth care.

- Cut down on caffeine and alcohol – which make stress worse.
- Try out various relaxation therapies and see which one works for you. Meditation and body-calming activities like yoga seem to help reduce the stress that aggravates habitual grinding.
- To relax clenched muscles before you go to bed or in the morning, apply a warm face cloth to the side of your face.
- Visit your dentist who will suggest either a single treatment or combination of treatments. This might include muscle relaxants to relax your jaw muscles. If that doesn't work you can be fitted with a special mouth guard which fits on to the lower or upper jaw and is worn at night. This removable plastic device prevents teeth from coming together, stopping further damage to your teeth. It may also stop the urge to grind. The idea is that it reprogrammes the part of your brain that controls movement, so that your jaw doesn't receive the signal to start grinding. To treat the damage caused by more serious cases of grinding, your dentist may reshape your biting surfaces with crowns or inlays.

'Be true to your teeth and they won't be false to you.'
SOUPY SALES, US TV presenter

Defining idea…

59

How did it go?

Q **My dentist is giving me a night guard to wear at night, but it hasn't stopped me grinding my teeth during the day. Surely, this means the problem isn't solved, doesn't it?**

A   *True – you can't solve teeth grinding with a night guard – it's simply masking the problem. You need to work out the sources of your stress and develop a plan to deal with them. This may include better time management and strategies like learning to say no plus having a variety of relaxation techniques to draw upon. Failing that, you may need to seek counselling.*

Q **I'm finding it difficult to work out when an episode of teeth grinding is about to come on. Is there anything I can do to help spot and control it?**

A   *A complementary practice called biofeedback training might be worth investigating. Biofeedback techniques help train people to control their involuntary nervous system with learned responses to fluctuating body conditions. It's particularly useful for stress-related conditions and you can use it to help control teeth grinding. During a training session, a monitoring system emits a sound to alert you when you're grinding your teeth. You then learn to recognise what's happening to your body. After this, you're taught breathing patterns and relaxation exercises that you can use whenever you feel the urge to grind.*

Q **My son has bruxism. Will he grow out of it?**

A   *Chances are, he will. Children with bruxism usually stop grinding their teeth before they reach adulthood. Most adults with the condition get it for the first time when they're teenagers – and it rarely begins after the age of 40.*

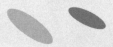

14

Cry babies

When you had your baby, you knew you'd be up and about in the middle of the night for night-time feeds. But your manual said it would all be over by four months. How wrong it was.

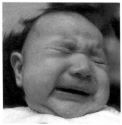

Many young children, understandably unfamiliar with these manuals, take years to get the message about sleeping through the night. This is why so many of us find ourselves treading the boards in the small hours — for months on end — the idea of unbroken sleep a dim and distant memory.

Some babies go to sleep like angels, but develop the habit of waking in the middle of the night at around ten months old. They've just learned that things still exist even when out of sight. When they wake up in the night, they now know that you must be nearby, so they call for you. The problem often goes away when the child

Here's an idea for you... **Prevent night-time waking in the first place by training your baby when she's very young. By three or four months, make it a habit to put your baby down to sleep when she's drowsy but not yet fully asleep. That way, she won't develop a habit of having to be held by you each time she wakes in the middle of the night.**

begins to walk, then reappears around 18 months, as problems of separation normally become a bit worse. Not all babies go through these phases, but many do.

Sometimes children wake up because as babies they never learned how to fall asleep on their own. Babies can become dependent on being held, sung to, rocked, breastfed, given a bottle, or even driven in a car in order to fall asleep. Our daughter wouldn't go to sleep unless I rocked her gently while my husband played 70s rock classics on his guitar. When she was asleep in my arms, I'd place her ever so slowly and carefully into her cot – but if the impact with the mattress wasn't completely smooth she'd wake up with a piercing cry and we'd have to start the process all over again.

If you always hold or rock your baby until he is completely asleep, rather than putting him down in the crib when he is drowsy but still a little bit awake, your baby develops a habit of having to be in your arms before he can fall asleep. Your baby associates the feeling of being held with the process of falling to sleep. Without the holding, he simply can't fall asleep. And if you give your baby a bottle to fall asleep with, he may come to rely on that as a trigger for sleep. Soon you'll find yourself fixing bottles two or three times a night.

An illness can also set you back. Your child may have been sleeping through the night for months, but then they get an ear infection, a cold or start teething. Your child may get used to being comforted at night so once the pain has gone he may whimper in the hope of some attention. Can you blame them? When they have been picked up and treated to company and a snack for several nights they learn to rouse themselves from half awake to wide awake to have more fun.

Are you prepared to follow a routine and be consistent? If so, your child can learn to sleep through the night – just follow the strategies in IDEA 27, *No baby no cry*.

Try another idea…

If you don't deal with night-time wakings, the problem probably won't go away – some 10% of four-year-olds still wake up at night. Soon your child will start coming into your own bed and before you know it, the family is playing musical beds. I know plenty of families where the dad either ends up on his own under his daughter's Barbie duvet cover or downstairs on the sofa, while mum is sandwiched between two fidgety young children.

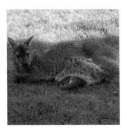

'*People who say they sleep like a baby usually don't have one.*'

Reverend LEO J BURKE

Defining idea…

How did it go?

Q Why do children wake up at night?

A   *Waking up at night is normal – everyone wakes up three or four times – what is not normal is being unable to get yourself back to sleep. If your child is always tended to when she wakes during the night, she won't learn to fall back to sleep on her own and will stay awake until your provide her with the comfort she's come to expect – whether that's in the form of a bottle, a dummy, cuddles and lullabies or a place beside you in bed.*

Q Our three-year-old son has been sleeping through for nearly two years. Why has he suddenly starting waking up and crying – often three or four times a night?

A   *A sudden change in sleeping habits could point to a health problem such as an allergy, asthma, or a pain like earache or teething. Loud snoring or pauses in breathing may mean he has obstructive sleep apnoea caused by enlarged adenoids or tonsils. Check these out with your doctor.*

Q Ever since my daughter started school she's been waking up in the night – could there be a connection?

A   *This sounds like stress-related waking which many children suffer after a big change like a new school, nanny, house or sibling. Give your daughter extra love and attention during the day and arrange to spend as much fun time with her as possible until she's feeling more secure. When you tuck her in, relieve any fears that she may have about school. If she wakes up in the middle of the night, go to her and reassure her, but don't stay for more than a few minutes – you don't want it to become a habit.*

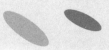

15

Ahhhhhh!!

Scary monsters or your mother in law ... don't let nightmares and night terrors ruin your sleep.

You're desperately trying to run, but your legs have got lead weights attached to them. You're being chased by your old history teacher who's wearing a black mask and carrying a gun — you've got to get away. Suddenly you cry out 'No!' and find yourself sitting up in bed, your heart thumping, unable to get back to sleep.

Most of us have experienced nightmares at one time or another. They're very common in children – particularly between the ages of three and four and seven and eight – and still about 5–10% of adults get them once a month. You'll normally have your nightmare during the second half of the night when you're in REM (dream) sleep. Suddenly you'll be woken up by a particularly harrowing episode – just before you're shot or pushed over the cliff, for instance. You'll be scared,

Here's an idea for you...

If you have had a particular nightmare more than once, recall it in as much detail as you can, and write it down. Think about how you could change the outcome of the dream. For instance, if you're being chased, stop running. Turn to face the pursuer and reason with the character or animal. If you're falling, relax and allow yourself to land: the old wives' tale is false – you will not really die if you hit the ground. Or transform falling into flying. Then find a time and place where you can be alone for 10–20 minutes. In a comfortable position, close your eyes, relax and visualise the new outcome of your dream. When the imagined dream has ended, write it down. The idea is that when you have the same dream again it will have your new ending. If it doesn't work first time, try it a few times.

anxious, very alert and will probably be able to recall your nightmare in great detail. Then you'll have trouble getting back to sleep.

They're different from night terrors, which suddenly appear out of deep non-dreaming sleep and normally happen in the first half of the night. In a night terror, you'll sit up suddenly and scream – but you probably won't wake up even though, rather scarily for your bed partner, your eyes might be wide open. You might sweat and your heart rate could shoot up three times its normal rate – much higher than with nightmares. Amazingly, you'll probably have no memory of it in the morning, just a vague sense of frightening images. Even if you are woken up when you're having a night terror, you won't be able to recall what happened – although studies have shown non-REM dreams are repetitive and thought-like, with little imagery – obsessively returning to a suspicion you left your mobile phone somewhere, for example.

ACTION PLAN

After you've had a nightmare, write down any factors that may have contributed to the bad dream. What did you eat yesterday? Did you have any alcohol? Are you stressed? Did you go to bed at a different time from usual? Did you watch a scary film? Are you ill or are you taking medication? All these factors can influence what you dream about.

Fatty and spicy food as well as cheese are thought to increase the chance of night-mares. Stress is also a common trigger – whether it's work, financial difficulties, moving house, relationship problems, bereavement or even pregnancy. Drinking and medication increase the risk, too. The same factors influence night terrors – particularly stress and being overtired.

If you find what's causing the nightmares or night terrors, deal with the trigger. That said, it's not always as easy as giving up cheese before bedtime and avoiding late night horror films. Sometimes you won't know the cause. With nightmares, talking through them – even drawing images from them – can help. With night terrors, talking often doesn't help because you can't remember the content. If they're really severe and happen often, talk to your doctor about medication such as the tranquil-liser diazepam.

'I don't use drugs, my dreams are frightening enough.'
Artist MC ESCHER

Defining idea…

Train yourself to influence your dreams in IDEA 28, *Dreamworks* – you can not only learn to stop nightmares but use your dreams to deal with stress.

Try another idea…

How did
it go?

Q   **The other day my son started crying and screaming in his sleep. He was thrashing around, with his eyes open, but was sleeping calmly again after about five minutes. Was this a nightmare?**

A   *No it sounds like a night terror. Though they're frightening to witness, they're not a cause for concern. There's little you can do when one strikes. Don't hug him or hold him down – it'll make him agitated and he'll probably push you away. And don't try to wake him up – this will only prolong it. Don't even mention it the next day – he won't remember it so it won't help. If your son has a nightmare, however, encourage him to talk about it. Children's nightmares are normally one way of dealing with everyday fears and problems. And with a nightmare, when your child wakes up, give him lots of hugs and reassure him he's safe.*

Q   **Are nightmares hereditary?**

A   *No, not particularly. But night terrors tend to run in families and usually start before the age of ten.*

Q   **Why does drinking alcohol increase the risk of nightmares?**

A   *If you go to sleep drunk, you may sleep quite soundly, but dream little, until five or six hours into sleep. Then, the alcohol's effect has mostly worn off and your brain is prepared to make up for the lost REM time. So you'll dream more intensely than usual and may well get nightmares. Some drugs and medications work in the same way – they suppress REM sleep so you get a double whammy when the drug wears off.*

16

Wet, wet, wet!

It's 3a.m. and you hear your child cry out. You go to his bedroom in a daze, remove the wet sheet, wipe down the plastic undersheet and put on a new sheet; then you change his pyjamas, give him a kiss and make your way back to bed – via the laundry basket.

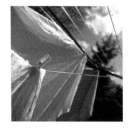

Now you're awake, unable to get back to sleep worrying about the bedwetting and all those other little niggles that have built up over the day. This has happened every night for the past month …

Almost half of all children still wet the bed at age three. In fact, most experts consider bedwetting normal until age six, when only 12% of kids still wet the bed. So why do some take so much longer to stay dry at night? For a start, bedwetting is hereditary – more than a quarter of kids whose parents were both bedwetters end up the same. And most seem to be very deep sleepers. Whereas other children wake up when they sense that their bladders are full, your child may simply have difficulty rousing. And some kids just need to wee more at night – maybe due to a smaller-than-average bladder.

Here's an idea for you... **Some experts suggest getting your child to take responsibility by helping with the wet sheets and putting on a new one. This is not a punishment. The idea is that children will often feel better by helping with the cleaning-up process.**

So what should you do? For a start, if your child isn't ready to sleep without night nappies, don't force him. All of you will sleep better if your child stays in nappies at night until he's ready to stay dry. If he sometimes wakes up dry or his nappy is barely damp in the morning instead of looking like a water-filled balloon, he may be ready to try. But if after a few weeks your child wets the bed frequently, you may have to put him back in nappies or disposable training pants. Tell him in a reassuring way that his body isn't ready to stay dry at night yet, and try again in a few months.

Even if your child is over six, his bedwetting will probably resolve itself naturally – with the right encouragement, support and positive reinforcement. Offering incentives like a small treat if they wake up dry can work. Whatever you do, don't punish your child for bedwetting. This will make him feel bad and will probably make the problem worse. No one wets the bed on purpose – after all, it's often embarrassing and uncomfortable. Would you like to wake up in a damp pool wearing cold, soggy pyjamas?

Whatever you do, don't make your child feel like their problem is some terrible family secret that should never be spoken about. Reassure them that it's a common problem. And tell them about other family members who used to be wet but are now dry. Also explain the condition to them – buy a book aimed at children about bedwetting. The more they know about the condition, the more likely they'll be able to overcome it.

If your child is over six, he could try a buzzer alarm – a device which wakes your child when he wets. This eventually teaches him to wake when he needs to go. You may need to get your doctor to refer you to a sleep expert, however, to learn how to use it properly. Your doctor may also prescribe medications such as anti-diuretic hormones that can be sprayed up the nostrils before bed to stop the urge to go to the toilet. However, behavioural techniques, such as the buzzer alarm, are thought to work best.

Is your child waking up in the night even when she's not wet? Take a look at IDEA 27, _No baby no cry_, to find out how to teach your child to go to sleep on her own again.

Try another idea…

'_All kids need is a little help, a little hope and somebody who believes in them._'

EARVIN 'MAGIC' JOHNSON

Defining idea…

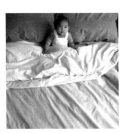
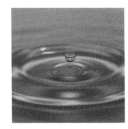
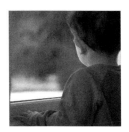

How did it go?

Q   My daughter often wets the bed at home, but when she stays at her grandma's house she's always dry in the morning. Why is this?

A   *Some children are drier when sleeping at a friend's or relative's home, but always wet in their own bed. Perhaps they do not sleep quite as deeply in a strange bed. This is especially frustrating for the child and parents. However, it's an excellent sign that the child should be able to be cured. These children may be consciously or subconsciously thinking about staying dry through the night when they are away from home. This kind of mental imagery can help.*

Q   Should I put my child on the toilet in the night to stop her wetting the bed?

A   *Most parents have tried waking their children up during the night to go to the toilet but often they are still wet in the morning. The problem is, it won't teach your child to go to the toilet herself – it could also wake her up and cause her distress. She needs to learn how to sleep through the night or wake up on her own. Another popular technique is to avoid giving your child fluids in the evening. This often makes no difference – your child will probably still be wet the next morning – and she'll be thirsty all night. That said, don't give your child caffeinated drinks like coke before bed.*

17

On the move

Odd things happen when there's a sleepwalker in the house – don't be surprised if you wake up to find the sofa cushions in the bath or that all those luxury Belgian chocolates have mysteriously disappeared ...

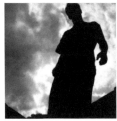

About 10–15% of us have been sleepwalking at some point in our lives – probably when we were children – and it's equally common in men and women. Here's how to spot the signs ...

When you sleepwalk you get out of bed and start to walk, then often perform acts in a robot-like way – anything from pacing the room to getting dressed and making yourself a cheese and ham sandwich. Most of the time sleepwalking isn't dangerous unless you go outside or turn on an appliance. And if you've walked a long time, you could go back to sleep somewhere other than bed. Next morning, it will come as a complete surprise when someone tells you of your night-time wanderings. Unless you wake up in the bath, of course.

Here's an idea for you... **If one of your family is sleepwalking, just gently guide them back to bed. Sleepwalkers who are suddenly woken up may be upset and have trouble falling asleep again. If the sleepwalker is in a dangerous situation, then you need to take some safety measures – particularly if the sleepwalker is a child. You should keep doors and windows closed and locked. This is especially important if you live in a flat. If necessary, your child may have to sleep on the ground floor of your home.**

HOW DOES IT HAPPEN?

It happens when parts of the brain are asleep and other parts of the brain – those that control walking and other physical activities – are in some way awake. You'd think that sleepwalking would happen during REM (dream sleep), but it actually occurs most often during very deep sleep, which takes place most often in the first third of the night. This is when the part of the brain that deals with thinking and alertness is asleep.

WHO SUFFERS?

You're more likely to sleepwalk if you're sleep deprived as you fall into a deep sleep more quickly. Some people say that the hormonal ups and downs of puberty, being pregnant and even having your period increase the chances of sleepwalking too. Stress is also a trigger – perhaps because your body finds it difficult to rest – and drinking alcohol can also lead to sleepwalking.

Children are most likely to sleepwalk as they spend more of the night in deep sleep when sleepwalking generally occurs. If your child sleepwalks, it's likely you or a member of you family also did so when you were children. The good news is that children tend to grow out of it. If you started sleepwalking after the age of nine, however, there's a higher chance you'll still be sleep-walking in adulthood.

Adult sleepwalking is more serious as it's often more extreme, and you're more likely to hurt yourself. One study of adult sleepwalkers found that 19% had been injured while sleepwalking. In the US, sleepwalkers are not allowed in the armed services, partly because of the threat they pose to themselves and others when they have access to dangerous equipment (such as weapons) and are unaware of what they are doing when they sleepwalk.

Do you also suffer nightmares or night terrors? Check out IDEA 15, *Ahhhhhh!* where you'll find out the difference between the two and learn how to deal with them.

Try another idea...

HOW IS IT TREATED?

If sleepwalking is not causing any problems and happens only occasionally, then nothing needs to be done. If it's getting you down, you need to tackle the cause. If it's triggered by alcohol, cut down and try not to drink after ten o'clock. If you're sleep deprived or stressed, deal with these, then the sleepwalking will probably stop. See your doctor about stress management techniques, counselling and relaxation exercises. The complementary therapies biofeedback, which teaches you to control various body functions, and hypnosis have been successful for sleepwalkers. As a last resort, talk to your doctor about drugs such as benzodiazepines, which can treat sleepwalk-ing by relaxing your muscles and preventing movement.

'People in a state of automatism don't have access to their full range of beliefs and desires, so it seems justifiable to excuse them.'
Philosopher NEIL LEVY
(University of Melbourne)

Defining idea...

How did
it go?

Q   Are sleepwalkers just acting out their dreams?

A   *No, acting out dreams is another condition called REM sleep disorder. Normally REM – rapid eye-movement – sleep, when you're most likely to dream,
is accompanied by paralysis, which protects us from acting out our dream. But
people with REM sleep disorder haven't got the chemical which stops them
acting out their dreams. These dreams are often physical or violent involving fighting, chasing or attacking and bed partners are often injured. Unlike
sleepwalkers, the sufferer doesn't normally leave the bed area.*

Q   How long do people sleepwalk for?

A   *Episodes usually last from one to five minutes, but may last up to an hour.*

Q   How do I know if I sleepwalk?

A   *First signs could be waking up with unexplained bruises, things left in the
wrong place and daytime tiredness. If in doubt get your partner or friend
to keep watch one night or ask your doctor to refer you to a sleep clinic.*

Q   Are you responsible for what happens when you sleepwalk?

A   *Strictly speaking, no, as you are not conscious. The husband of a sleepwalking Australian woman who left her house and had sex with strangers
for several months was very understanding when he found out. She was
eventually treated successfully by sleep medicine experts. And American
Ken Parks was acquitted of murder because he was sleepwalking at the
time. He drove 23 kilometres to his in-laws' house where he strangled his
father-in-law unconscious, and stabbed his mother-in-law to death.*

18

Open all hours

Working the overnight shift? How to make sure you're getting enough sleep.

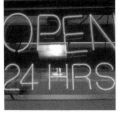

Millions of people now work during a time normally reserved for sleep in industries that never shut down. Just how does the body clock cope?

It's 4 o'clock in the morning in the world that never sleeps. You can do your weekly shop, buy an airline ticket or check your bank account over the phone if you wish while people all over the world are working in call centers and supermarkets to make this possible.

Shiftwork now accounts for nearly a quarter of all workers and keeps increasing with the demands of our 24/7 consumer society. Many factories now run 24 hours a day – and businesses that work all night include radio and TV stations, grocery shops and supermarkets and petrol stations as well as all the companies that service those businesses. Then there's the increasing number of call centres from computer support to advice on how to mend your dishwasher which employ people who are ready to help you any time, any day.

Here's an idea for you... **Unhappy with your work–life balance? Work out if the advantages of your job are worth the trade-off. Make a list of your values and priorities. Then cross off the items on your list that are not really all that important to you. Once you're down to two or three important values, you can see whether your lifestyle and your life fit with those values. If one of your priorities is to see your children and your work makes this impossible, then maybe you should change your lifestyle and schedule. Think about changing shifts. If that's not possible consider another job, retraining or going part time until you find something else.**

The problem with the increase in shift work is the effect on people's body clocks. When you stay awake at night you're fighting your body clock which is telling you to go to sleep. It's like getting jet lag every few days and can mean feeling groggy and tired all week. Many of the health and other problems associated with shift work are similar to those suffering from sleep deprivation – higher risk of accidents and errors at work, increased chance of heart disease and poor concentration.

SHIFT WORK SOLUTIONS

You need to work out if you're getting the right amount of sleep so you can be healthy, and not endanger yourself or others. These tips might help.

■   As far as you can, choose shifts that work with your body clock. If you're a night owl you're not going to have much problem staying awake at night – so an evening and night shift would be best for you. If you're a lark, you'll be happy to start work at 6a.m., but would probably not be able to cope with a night shift.

- At work, don't leave the boring stuff until the end of the day – you might find it difficult to finish. And if you're getting sleepy at the end of your shift, either go for a short break or ask one of your colleagues to step in for you – particularly if the consequences of making an error would be great such as when operating heavy machinery or in air traffic control. You will do the same for them.
- If you finish your shift in the day, wear wraparound sunglasses – particularly if it's sunny – exposure to bright light in the morning may reset your body clock and make it difficult to sleep.
- Avoid heavy meals and alcohol before sleeping – having a big meal at breakfast time will make it harder to sleep.
- If you need to sleep during the day, make sure your home is sleep-friendly. Invest in heavy blinds to blackout the bedroom. Turn off the phone's ringer. Make sure your family know not to interrupt you. Tell your neighbours about your shift work so they can keep the noise down in the day. And remember to be friendly and appreciative.

'Dawn: When men of reason go to bed.'

AMBROSE BIERCE, US writer
(1842–1914)

Defining idea…

If you need to sleep in your bedroom during the day, it's worth finding ways to block noises from outside. Take a look at IDEA 39, *What a racket!* for soundproofing tips.

Try another idea…

Q   What type of shift work is easiest?

A   *Fixed shifts are best for establishing a regular sleep pattern and lifestyle. You have a regular schedule when you always work at the same times. With rotating schedules, you work a few days at one shift, have a few days off and then switch to another shift. So sometimes you're working days, sometimes evenings, sometimes nights and sometimes mornings. Some people have completely irregular shifts and others have split shifts where the workday is split by a few hours. Rotating shifts are better when they go clockwise – i.e., days, evenings, nights rather than the other way round.*

Q   Most of my colleagues are unhappy with the shift schedules. Would it be possible to change them?

A   *You may have to talk to your boss or your union, if you're in one, to see what compromises and changes can be made. If you're serious, compile a document detailing the impact of shift work schedules on the health and productivity of their workers. Check to see if similar industries have different schedules. Arm yourself with all the research and other materials you need to present your case. And for the best chance of a response, suggest a better shift schedule that would increase productivity and improve the health of the workers.*

Q   Would a nap stop me getting so tired at the end of a shift?

A   *Yes, a short 15–25 minute nap can dramatically improve your alertness. You have to make sure you don't nap for too long, though – you'll fall into deep sleep and wake up groggier. All you need is a quiet room and a few comfy chairs. Check to see if your company has a napping policy.*

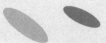

19

The jet set

Tanned, surrounded by unpacked bags and watching telly at 4.30a.m., there is no more tragic sight than the jet-lagged traveller attempting to put their life and their sleep pattern back on track.

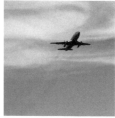

Whether you're starting your holiday or returning to work the morning after you get back, here's how to minimise the effects of time-zone hopping.

You get jet lag when you travel across time zones so fast that your body doesn't have time to adjust to the new day and night cues. The problem is you're messing with your internal body clock – which tells you when to sleep and when to be awake – and this takes a while to adjust to local time zones. On some long-haul flights, your jet lag can last anything from two to five days. With symptoms similar to those of a terrible hangover – tiredness during the day, inability to sleep at night, headache, diarrhoea – jet lag could easily put you off air travel altogether. Hopefully, these tips from airline crews can soften the blow. Happy holidays!

Here's an idea for you... **Apply a few drops of essential oil of tangerine, bergamot or lemon oil to the inside of your wrist or behind your ears to pep you up once you've arrived. Or unwind with lavender or clary sage after a long flight.**

- *Find the best time to fly.* Look at the differences in time zones, the direction you're travelling in, and work out the best time to travel to minimise the effects. When you fly east you lose time and your day becomes shorter, while by flying west you gain time and your day becomes longer. So an overnight flight is best if you're travelling east, a day flight if going west. Confused? Ask a mathematician.

- *Start training for your new time zone.* When going on long-haul flights, airline crews get up an hour earlier each day for a week before departure. If you're heading west, try to go to bed and get up an hour later each day. If you're going east go to bed earlier than usual.

- *Change your watch to your destination time as soon as your plane takes off.* This will help get your mind thinking in the new time and, psychologically, it will help your body to adapt itself to a different time zone.

- *Be flight smart.* Try to sleep at the new times on the plane. If you need to keep yourself awake, do crossword puzzles or listen to stimulating music. You could engage in conversation with the person next to you but there's always the risk he'll be a financial adviser who spends the entire flight trying to sell you life insurance. Don't read a novel or watch the video – they're guaranteed to send you into a slumber. And try to get a seat on the side that will get most sunlight during the flight. If you need to sleep, buy ear plugs. A sleeping pill for a night or two before the flight may make it easier to sleep on the plane.

- *Keep on the move.* During the flight, try to walk around as much as you can and, when sitting down, flex and extend your ankles to increase circulation. This will also help prevent swollen ankles and muscle stiffness. When you reach your destination, half an hour of exercise will keep you alert for up to two hours. Don't be tempted to perform star jumps in the baggage reclaim lounge, though – being escorted out of the airport by security is not a great start to any holiday. Just go for a brisk walk once you've dropped off your luggage.

- *Adjust your daylight exposure as soon as you arrive.* When you arrive in the new time zone, adjust your sleep schedule straight away to the local time. So if you arrive in the day but your body thinks it's night-time, go outside, get lots of sunshine and keep active to trick your body into staying awake (remember dark triggers sleep-inducing melatonin). Eat your meals at the local time, too. Try not to go to bed until it is bedtime in the local time zone. If you have to, take a 20-minute nap to help you get through the day.

If you're going to be driving after a long flight, make sure you stay alert at the wheel – take the advice in IDEA 20, *Dozy driving*, before you set off.

Try another idea…

'I love to travel but I hate to arrive.'

ALBERT EINSTEIN

Defining idea…

Q   Will drinking on the flight make any difference?

A   Yes, sorry – if you want to be perky when you arrive say no to that gin and tonic. Flying dehydrates you and alcohol will emphasise the effect, making you parched and tired. Drink plenty of water, not fizzy drinks – flying causes gases in your gut to expand so fizzy drinks make you even more bloated.

Q   When I get to my holiday destination, I'm going to have to stay awake much longer than normal to adjust to the new times. Is there anything I should eat?

A   Research shows that eating protein-rich food such as fish or eggs at break-fast and lunchtime helps you stay awake, while a dinner rich in carbohy-drates such as pasta and bread can make you sleepy.

Q   Which produces the worst symptoms – flying east or west?

A   Flying east because it shortens your day. You can feel anything from slight disorientation and fatigue to poor memory, insomnia, headaches, irritabil-ity and poor concentration.

Q   Do supplements help?

A   Some people take supplements before, during and after travelling. The most important ones include vitamins C and E. They help combat free radicals, harmful molecules in your body that increase as a result of atmos-pheric radiation in the cabin – which is thought to make jet lag worse. Some people swear by melatonin supplements. They're not available over the counter in all countries, but you can buy them on the internet.

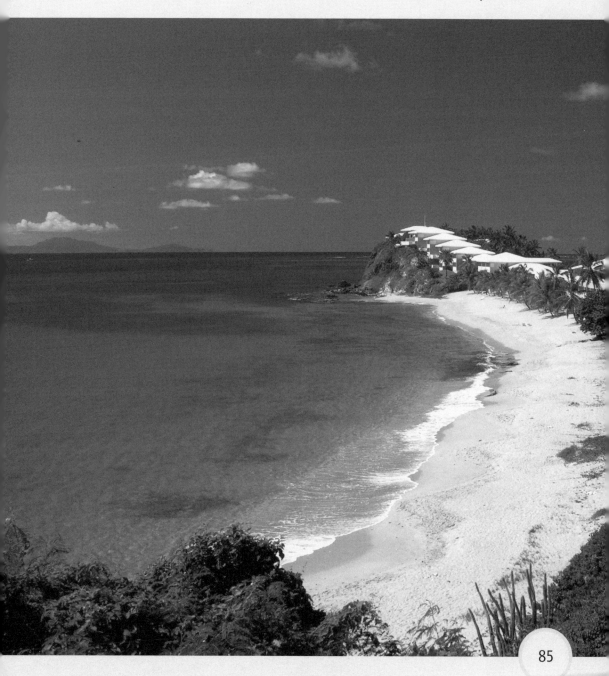

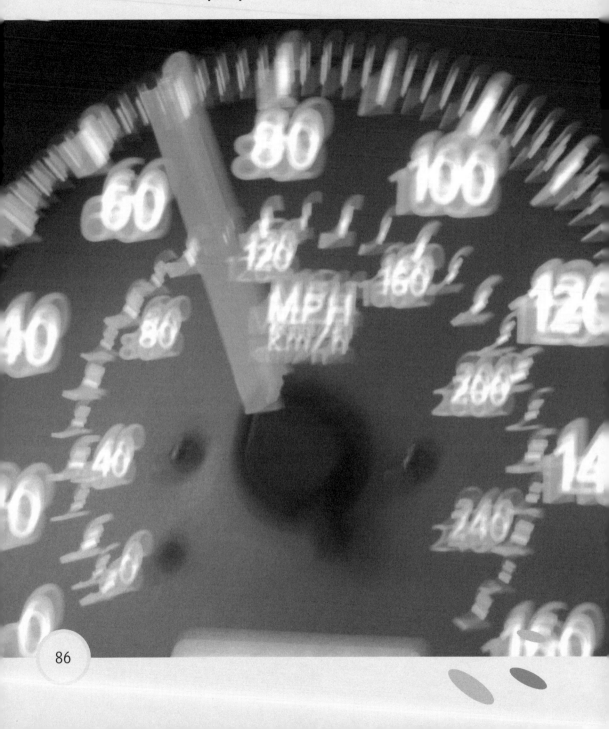

20

Dozy driving

Whether you're going on a long journey or you're simply on your way to work after a bad night's sleep, driving a car when you're tired can be fatal.

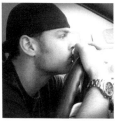

If you've had less than five hours' sleep, you'll drive like someone who's well over the legal drink-drive limit. It's not surprising then that one out of three car accidents is attributed to sleepiness.

Have you ever driven when tired? If you have, you're not alone – about 55% of drivers admit to driving when drowsy and a shocking two-thirds have admitted to falling asleep at the wheel at some point. Not only do tired drivers perform as poorly as drink drivers, studies show that drivers who have been awake for fifteen hours or more, are four times more likely to have an accident than a person who has had a good night's sleep. Another study showed that drivers who had had five hours' sleep had only a one in ten chance of staying fully awake on a long journey.

When you're sleepy everything slows down – from responding to the movements of the cars around you to making quick decisions in emergency situations. The

Here's an idea for you...

Stay alert with essential oils. Drop a few drops of stimulating oils such as lime, peppermint, lemongrass or black pepper onto a tissue, then every time you need a boost take an energising sniff. Alternatively, put your pick-me-up oils in an in-car vapouriser.

warning signs? You suddenly realise where you are and can't account for the last part of your journey, your thoughts are wondering, you're drifting over to the next lane, you're yawning or struggling to keep your eyes open or focused. If you've got any of these symptoms, you should stop as soon as it's safe and take a break. Ideally, you should only ever drive when well rested. In the real world, that's not always possible, so here's a few stay-awake strategies.

- *Don't take long trips on your own.* Travel with another person. Chatting will help keep you alert – unless your companion's favourite topic of conversation is molecular plant organisms. Even if it is, he could take over the wheel if you get tired. Some 82% of sleep-related crashes involved someone driving alone.
- *Play I spy.* If you've got children in the car, play games such as I spy or First one to see. Try the alphabet game where you have to spot something that starts with the letter A, then the letter B, all the way until Z. Or what about Guess who? where you have to think of a person or character, then everyone asks questions (you can only say yes or no) until someone works out who you are.
- *Avoid your sleepy times.* Between 12p.m. to 8a.m. and 1p.m. to 3p.m. are statistically the most dangerous time to drive. This is when you naturally feel most tired. This is because your body clock tells you to sleep regardless of whether you've had enough sleep. If you must drive during these times, be extra vigilant.

- *Take regular breaks*. If you're on a long journey, schedule regular stops every 150 km or two hours. Stop sooner if tired.
- *Drink caffeine*. OK I've said it's a no-no, but if you're tired at the wheel, it's a guaranteed way to pep you up. If you drive to work every morning, have a coffee just before you get in the car – this can be your daily quota. Research has found that a can of caffeinated energy drink or coffee can help you avoid the afternoon dip, and the effects last for about an hour and a half. Feeling dehydrated can also make you tired – so drink plenty of water.
- *Take a power nap*. When you're tired, pull over to a rest area, roll up the windows, lock the doors, and lie back for about 15 minutes (use an alarm clock to wake you up). Research shows that a 15-minute nap in the afternoon provides more rest than sleeping an extra 20 minutes in the morning.
- *Play music you love*. Stay away from snooze-inducing sounds such as classical tracks and slow ballads. Go for loud, fast-paced music that you can sing along to. You may catch people smirking as you belt out your favourite Beatles track at the top of your voice. But who cares?
- *Munch on energy snacks*. Being hungry will reduce your blood sugar levels and make you even more tired. So keep handy some dried apricots, nuts, raisins or dried banana.

Try another idea...

To find out more about the benefits of napping, take a look at IDEA 30, *Forty winks*. And for more on what to eat to stay alert throughout the day, check out IDEA 33, *Food for thought*.

Defining idea...

'The urge to continue driving despite acute feelings of sleepiness is rooted in a firm belief that "it won't happen to me".'
PERETZ LAVIE, professor of biological psychiatry

Q   Who's most likely to drive when tired?

A   *Young drivers, who tend to stay up later, have the most sleep-related
crashes, followed by shiftworkers and commercial drivers. People with an
untreated sleep disorder such as obstructive sleep apnoea can be 15 times
more likely to have an accident.*

Q   Does opening the window keep you awake?

A   *No – and don't rely on it. In fact the soothing sound of the wind can actually make you feel drowsy. That said, keeping the car too warm will make
you feel drowsy.*

Q   Can you drink alcohol the night before a long car journey?

A   *Not advisable, as it can interrupt your sleep and make you feel exhausted
the next morning. And never drink before you drive – particularly if you're
tired. Research shows that the effects of one beer on a person who has
had four hours' sleep is the equivalent of a six-pack on a well-rested
person.*

Q   Are there any exercises you can do to stay awake?

A   *It's probably not worth doing anything strenuous if you're speeding along
the motorway, but if traffic's at a standstill you could try this energising
move from the Japanese therapy* jin shin jyutsu: *hold the fourth and fifth
fingers of your right hand for as long as you can, then repeat on the other
hand.*

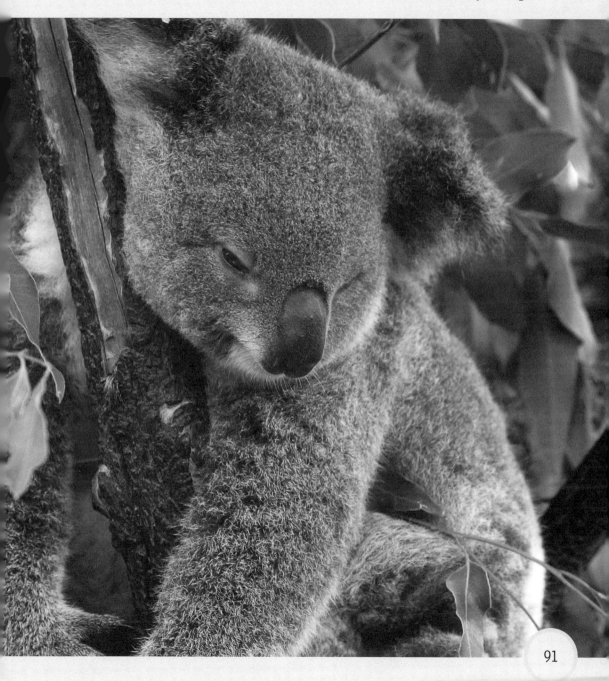

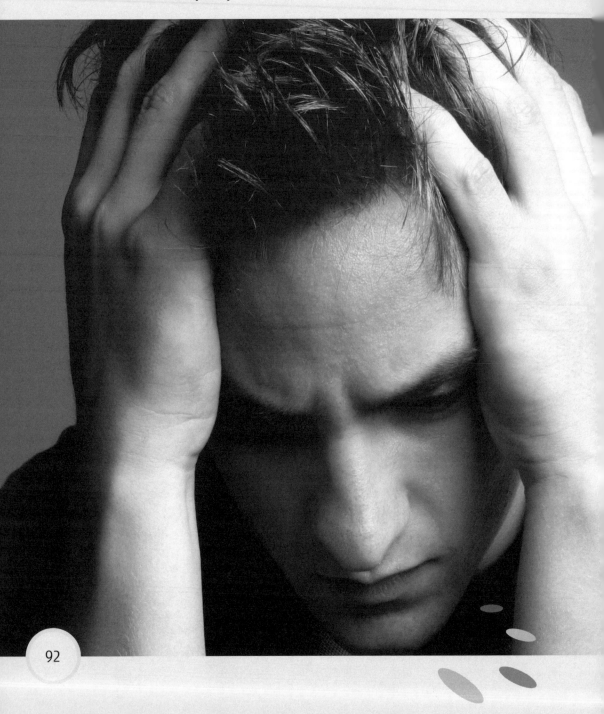

21

Snores you can't ignore

Do you sometimes go to bed early, yet wake up feeling groggy and are tired all day? If so, and you also snore, you could have sleep apnoea.

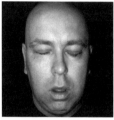

The scary thing about sleep apnoea is that you actually stop breathing for a bit. Unsurprisingly, this not only disrupts sleep but can lead to serious health problems ...

If your snoring is steady and regular it's probably nothing to worry about. But it could be a problem if you have loud, frequent bursts of snoring followed by quiet periods then a sudden gasping for air. These periods of silence mean that you're not breathing and can last from ten seconds to as long as two minutes. I can only imagine the fear felt by your loved one as they wait for you to start breathing again, trying to banish thoughts that you're only seconds away from death. This can happen hundreds of times a night although you'll have no recollection of it the next morning. The worst episodes are during dreaming (REM sleep). This is because people are paralysed in REM sleep so the muscles that keep the airway open are paralysed too.

Here's an idea for you... **Try the following experiment to help you understand what happens during an episode of sleep apnoea. Put your hand over your vacuum cleaner intake nozzle. Your hand blocks all air from getting through even though the vacuum cleaner is still applying suction in the same way that we still try to breathe. The vacuum cleaner will be straining now – just as your body would be.**

WHY YOU STOP BREATHING

Your throat closes and you cannot suck air into your lungs. This is because the muscles that hold your throat open when you're awake relax during sleep and allow it to narrow. So when your throat is partially closed or the muscles relax too much, every time you inhale you'll suck your throat until it's completely closed and air won't be able to pass at all. So how does breathing go back to normal? Rising carbon dioxide levels wake you up slightly, and this sends a signal from the brain to the throat muscles that enlarge the airway to open up – so breathing starts again, often with a loud snort or gasp.

As you can imagine, this is not a healthy state of affairs. When you stop breathing, the level of oxygen in the blood goes down and the level of carbon dioxide goes up. The low blood oxygen level forces the heart to work harder which changes your heart rate and may increase blood pressure. A study in Israel found that sufferers were more likely to have hardened arteries, which increases the risk of heart disease and strokes.

The rise in carbon dioxide levels also affect circulation, particularly the circulation of your brain. If you're regularly waking up with headaches, this is probably why. And then, of course, you're less alert in the day. A research team from Spain says that people with sleep apnoea are seven times more likely to crash than other drivers.

WHAT TRIGGERS IT?

As with snoring, smoking, drinking alcohol and being overweight can bring it on. In fact, alcohol can turn snoring into apnoea. Someone who normally only snores may actually stop breathing while sleeping after drinking even small amounts of alcohol. About 75% of sleep apnoea patients are overweight – and often symptoms only start after you gain a lot of weight. This is why it's common during pregnancy when it has to be treated seriously as it can affect the baby. If the blood level of oxygen is too low in the mother when she sleeps, it will be too low for the baby. There's evidence that babies can be smaller as a result.

Sleep apnoea can also be caused by a blockage in the nose or throat such as a short jaw, large tonsils or adenoids, swollen nasal passages from allergies or a tongue that is too far back.

Not everyone who snores has apnoea and not everyone with apnoea necessarily snores – although by far the majority do. Often symptoms come on so slowly that apnoea is not spotted until something dramatic happens. This could include nodding off inappropriately in the day while driving and personality changes such as irritability and inability to concentrate.

'Laugh and the world laughs with you. Snore and you sleep alone.'

ANTHONY BURGESS

Defining idea…

From self-help strategies to machines that open up the airways, turn to IDEA 25, *Breathe easy*, for how to treat sleep apnoea.

Try another idea…

Q **If I was waking in the night and having all these symptoms, wouldn't I be aware of it?**

A *Amazingly, most people with sleep apnoea have no idea they're waking to breathe many times during the night. Many people don't realise they have it and even think they're good sleepers. It's not until they see and hear themselves at a sleep clinic that they realise they have a problem. Although it's easy to get used to these slight arousals, it's enough to disrupt your night's sleep so you don't get enough deep sleep or REM sleep.*

Q **Who's most likely to suffer?**

A *It affects about 3% of people overall and is more common in men – at the age of 30 men are five times more likely than women to develop sleep apnoea in the next ten years. But over the age of 50 it's more common in women – they're three times more likely to have sleep apnoea after meno-pause. This is because of the drop in female hormones that protect women against apnoea – and that many women put on weight at this time.*

Q **When do you go to the doctor?**

A *If you stop breathing for more than ten seconds at a time more than ten times an hour and you're feeling excessively tired in the day.*

Q **Why does apnoea only happen when you're asleep?**

A *When you sleep, the muscle tone in your upper airway relaxes and this causes the airway to collapse. During the day you have enough muscle tone to keep the airway open to breathe normally.*

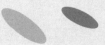

22

Say no to stress

Calm-down strategies to stop night-time niggles.

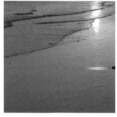

Whatever's keeping you up at night — thoughts of strangling your boss who's giving you a hard time at work or an inability to stop thinking about all those things you didn't manage to do today — stressbusting techniques can help. These will help control your stress before it spirals out of control ...

Once you've made a stress diary of the people and events that trigger your stress, talk through it with a good friend or your partner – even the act of discussing things often makes you feel better. Ask for impartial advice as to how to ease the problems that you've discovered. And once you know your stress triggers, try to nip them in the bud. Changing your routine can help. For instance, a friend of mine who felt stressed every time he saw the iron on Sunday night now irons his shirts in the week. This has stopped him associating ironing with the start of a new week. And

Here's an idea for you... **To banish stress-related headaches and insomnia, try hand reflexology. Stretch out your right hand and, with your left thumb, apply pressure from the base of your hand and work your way up to the top of your thumb tip. Repeat ten times. Alternatively, use scent to improve your mood. Drip a few drops of some of the following aromatherapy oils on a tissue to sniff when you feel stress levels rising: jasmine, neroli, lavender, chamomile, vetiver or clary sage.**

learn a few relaxation or breathing exercises which you can perform as soon as your stress levels start to rise. And if you know your stress trigger, you can calm yourself beforehand.

There's nothing more stressful than being disorganised, so get your life in order. If you've got a list of jobs that need doing, set yourself two tasks and make sure you do them. Then whatever else the day throws at you, at least you'll have achieved something. For real satisfaction, choose two of the things that keep finding their way to the bottom of your list. Chances are they're the things that whirr through your mind in the middle of the night preventing you from going back to sleep.

And learn to slow down – don't try to juggle two or more tasks at once. Research shows that people who patiently complete one task at a time, with undivided attention have more calm energy than those who try to do too many things at once. Juggling projects increase tensions, which lowers energy. So allow yourself plenty of time to complete a task – even if it means delegating other jobs or getting less done that day. Some people swear by doing the worst task first – the theory is that once this is out of the way, everything else will seem easier.

Another general stress reliever is to plan breaks in your day. Get up 15 minutes earlier than you think you need to and prepare for the day without rushing. You'll leave the house in a calmer, more positive mood. And try to have 20 minutes in the morning and afternoon that is exclusively 'your' time, in which you can do whatever you want, even if it is simply sitting doing nothing.

Remember that the way you look at what's going on around you has a major affect on how good you feel about yourself and how stressed you are. When you think positively, you are likely to be calmer and more relaxed. For example if you say to yourself 'I can do this' or 'I'm good at making decisions' you're encouraging yourself and will feel less stressed. Negative self-talk such as 'This is terrible' and 'I'm hopeless' will do the opposite and reduce your confidence. Pay attention to your self-talk and keep it positive.

Finally, don't let a work problem such as bullying get out of control. Keep a written record of all the incidents involving the bully so you can see if a pattern emerges. Bullies usually strike when they're trying to cover up their own incompetence. Keep copies of all letters and emails written by the bully and record all criticisms in writing. Then you can take up the matter with management and get a copy of your employer's bullying and harassment policy.

A great way to manage stress is to perform a regular relaxation technique. To find out how easy it is to meditate, check out IDEA 43, *Ommmm ...* and to pick up some calming poses, go to IDEA 42, *Say yes to yoga.*

Try another idea...

'For fast-acting relief, try slowing down.'

LILY TOMLIN,
actress and comedienne

Defining idea...

99

How did
it go?

Q **I'm always in a bad mood with my children and they always seem to be playing up. At the end of the day I feel stressed and that I've barely achieved anything. What can I do?**

A *First of all, take your time and try to enjoy your children. Most of your everyday activities will take longer when you have a child so give yourself extra time to avoid the feeling of being rushed. Your children will also react better when the pressure is off. And before getting cross with them, think about whether an issue is really worth worrying about. For example, you may decide that you need to intervene if your children are being unkind to each other, but that it's not worth taking a stand over whether plates are left in the sink or put in the dishwasher. Save your energy for issues which really matter to your family and let the little things go by.*

Q **Can you suggest any good stress reliever I could do in my lunch-time?**

A *Go for a walk. You do not have to be a gym freak to get the stress-beating benefits of exercise. Even 20 minutes of brisk walking three times a week will help to reduce stress as well as promoting restful sleep.*

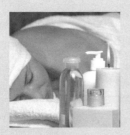

23

Sunday night insomnia

How to halt the Monday morning blues in its tracks.

Monday, if you're not careful, can reach into Sunday night with a grasping claw-like hand, starting a chain of panicky thoughts that eventually stop you falling asleep at night. What is supposed to be part of your weekend turns quickly into a painful rehearsal for the next day's challenges ...

The week ahead need not start till 9.30 Monday morning, if you take steps to keep that drawer full of unfinished work firmly shut until you're actually in a position to do something about it.

■ Don't lie in at the weekend. This is one of the reasons you feel more tired on a Monday morning. Your body clock gets resynchronised with the sleep-wake cycle every night and even small changes can affect it negatively. You should get up at the same time, even weekends, because every time you sleep in you delay

Here's an idea for you…

Save time and cut morning stress by preparing for work the night before. So wash and blow-dry your hair and lay out a clean, ironed outfit for the next day. If you've got children, lay out their clothes and bags.

the rise in your body temperature, which means you delay the time you're likely to get to sleep the following night.

- Tackle next week's issues. Sunday night is classically spent worrying about all those things you need to do but haven't … not forget your mum's birthday, get your mum's birthday present, pay final reminder gas bill, phone the plumber, work out where all your money's going … The problem is there's nothing you're going to be able to do at 11 p.m. on Sunday night so all you can do is punish yourself. Why not select a time every week either early in the day on Sunday or Saturday morning when you deal with troublesome thoughts. Write down all the things worrying you and come up with ways to tackle them. You should find it easier to sleep knowing that you have a strategy and that you're in control of the situation.

- Say no to Sunday roast. Eating a huge meal will deplete your energy. Being uncomfortably full promotes sluggishness and makes you desperate for an afternoon snooze. But if you do take a nap you'll find it harder to sleep that night, giving you a bad start to the week. Eat a light meal and go for a stroll an hour after eating to ward off lethargy.

- Give yourself a treat. One way of tackling Sunday insomnia is to use Sunday evening to plan a treat for Monday or Tuesday. This could be a meal out, going to the cinema or getting together with friends. Focusing on something positive will stop you dreading the following Monday morning.

- Don't binge drink. You're binging if you regularly have more than the recommended amount of alcohol at weekends – that's over two to three units a day for women or four for men (a unit is one small glass of wine, a pub measure of spirits or half a pint of lager or beer). Apart from giving you a draining hangover, drinking too much also makes you more likely to call in sick to work, have arguments or suffer accidents.

- Get the right balance. Don't bring work home at the weekend – it's guaranteed to make you feel as if you haven't had a break when you get back to work on Monday morning. If you can't get everything done during the week then you might be in the wrong job. You're either in a job that can't be done in the allotted time or you're not suited to it. Talk to your boss about how you can plan your time more efficiently or delegate some of your workload.

- If you're feeling restless on Sunday night, then get more active in the day. Inject your weekend activities with energy – instead of simply meeting friends for a lunchtime drink, do something physical. Try team sports which combine socialising with activity. You'll have more energy during the weekend and be more physically exhausted Sunday night, making it easier for you to drop off.

Try another idea…

If stress is affecting your sleep all week – not just on Sundays – take a look at IDEA 10, *All stressed out*! And then pick up some calm-down strategies in IDEA 22, *Say no to stress*.

Defining idea…

'It is better to sleep on things beforehand than lie awake about them afterward.'
BALTASAR GRACIAN,
Spanish philosopher (1601–58)

103

How did it go?

Q **Why do I always argue with my partner at the weekends? How can we stop going to bed on Sunday night in a bad mood with each other?**

A *If you're so busy during the week that you don't get a chance to discuss any problems with your partner, it can mean that when you get to the weekend you spend the whole time arguing with each other. If you still haven't made up by Sunday night, you won't be able to go to sleep because all those hurtful comments you hurled at each other are still whirring about in your head. To stop this happening, make sure that you schedule in an hour so in the week to talk over anything that's bothering you. This way you can resolve the issue before the weekend, leaving you both free to enjoy yourselves together.*

Q **The weekend never turns out how I want it to, so I'm dissatisfied and irritated when I attempt to go to sleep on Sunday night. Why do I always end up doing what other people want to do?**

A *Having to participate in chores or activities you don't want to do at the weekend can make you feel resentful, which is very draining. You need to learn to say no. This frees up your time so you can enjoy yourself more. If you find it hard to refuse, try this technique: say no in a neutral tone of voice, be polite but don't feel you have to give an excuse. You'll be surprised how easy it is once you've done it.*

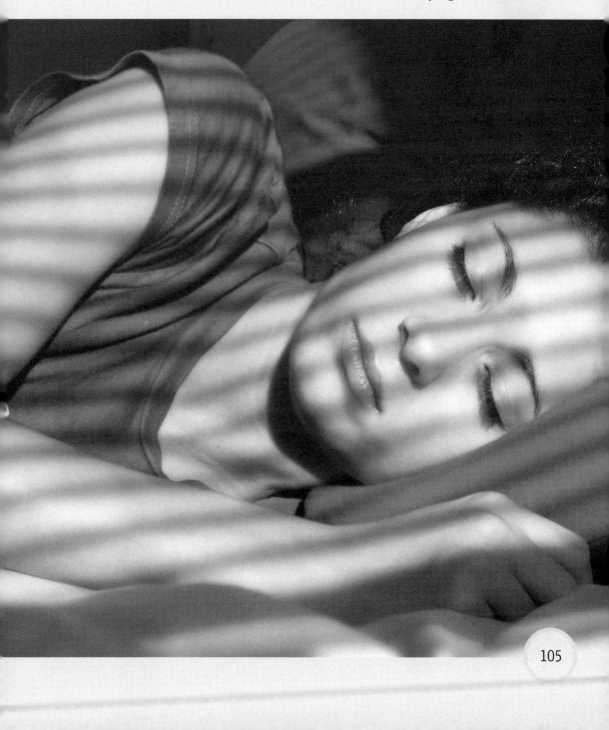

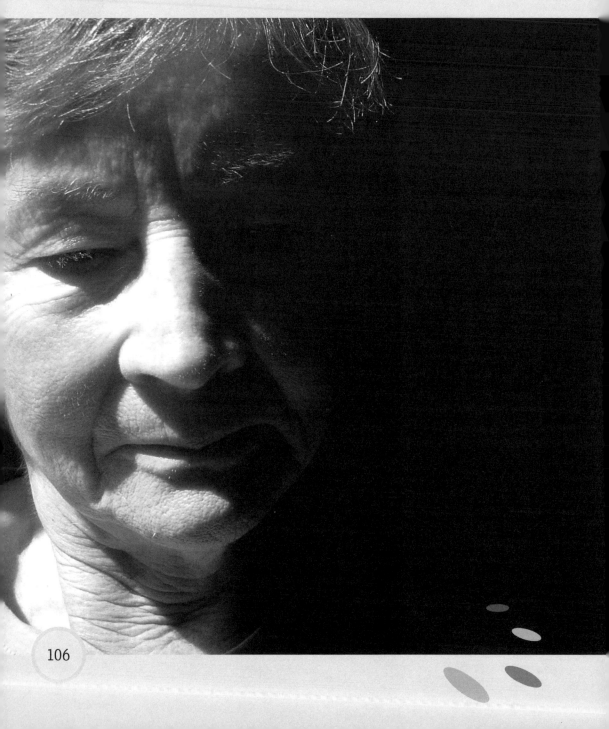

24

More than just the blues

If you're depressed, chances are you're not sleeping very well either. Tackle the depression, though, and the insomnia goes too.

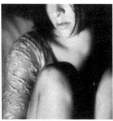

Statistics show that about one in five adults with insomnia have depression and three-quarters of all people with insomnia will have depression at some time in their lives. And 90% of people with depression have insomnia.

If you're depressed, you'll be sad or anxious pretty much all the time. You may be restless and irritable and cry for no reason. You'll have little interest in anything – including sex – and you'll feel drained. You'll have low self-esteem and fail to see the positive in anything. You might either sleep too much or too little. Similarly, your appetite may shoot up or you'll not be hungry at all. You could also get physical symptoms, such as stomach pains, headaches and rapid heartbeat. Most people get depressed now and again – it's only a problem if it doesn't go away and your sleep is still suffering.

Here's an idea for you...

Dwelling on past hurts will make you feel bitter and resentful, so savour your positive past. Every day for a whole week, set aside five minutes each morning and night to think about some of the loveliest things you've experienced. Research has shown that being positive helps you recover from psychological problems and emerge much stronger. It's also important to remember even though you can't control your past, you can determine your future. Take a pen and paper and imagine who and where you want to be, then work out what steps you need to take.

WHAT CAUSES IT?

It's often triggered by stress, bereavement, financial problems or difficult relationships and having a negative outlook makes you more prone as it makes you less able to cope. As a result, there'll be a drop in the key chemicals in your brain responsible for regulating mood – serotonin and noreinephrine. You need serotonin to produce your sleep-inducing melatonin, so it's inevitable your sleep will suffer.

WHAT'S THE TREATMENT?

Your doctor will give you an assessment to make sure you haven't got another underlying condition such as an underactive thyroid or anaemia which can also make you tired. He may prescribe antidepressants which affect the levels of your brain chemicals. There are more than 25 different types of antidepressants and your doctor will recommend one which is the right one for you. Selective serotonin reuptake inhibitors (SSRIs) like Prozac work by boosting serotonin levels. Others, such as amitriptylines, act as a sedative as well as increase serotonin. The most effective treatment, however, is some form of talking therapy on its own or combined with medication.

A counsellor or psychotherapist will help you get to the root of the problem. Once you've discovered why you're depressed and learned how to cope, your depression is less likely to come back. Psychoanalysts – one of the most common types of psychotherapist – often blame depression on an inability to deal with anger and a desperate need for approval. You'll have to delve deep into the past to resolve these issues – and this can take years. Cognitive therapists don't look to the past so much and believe depressed people are caught in a cycle of negative thinking and expect to fail. Your therapist will help change the way you think. Counselling can be useful if your depression is triggered by a specific problem such as a difficult relationship or dealing with the loss of a loved one.

Check out IDEA 22, *Say no to stress*, for tips on learning how to deal with stress, and for advice on using positive thinking to tackle your sleep problems, take a look at IDEA 32, *Mind power*.

Try another idea…

ARE YOU FEELING SAD?

If you start to feel low as soon as winter sets in you may have seasonal affective disorder (SAD) which is triggered by a lack of daylight. If you have a mild form, you'll feel slightly more tired and fed up in winter than at other times of the year. If it's more extreme, you'll sleep more, feel lethargic when you're awake and crave stodgy foods. Light goes in through the eye and travels to the part of the brain that controls mood, appetite, food and sex drive – so if you're not getting enough light these will be badly affected. Lack of light also makes you produce more melatonin, making you feel sleepy. The best treatment is light therapy where you're exposed to bright light from a lightbox for between 15 and 45 minutes a day. Your doctor may also prescribe the antidepressants SSRIs, which boost levels of the feelgood hormone serotonin.

'Noble deeds and hot baths are the best cures for depression.'
DODIE SMITH, English author (1896–1990)

Defining idea…

109

Q **Are there any natural remedies for depression?**

A *St John's wort has been used for centuries to treat depression and some studies have suggested it's just as effective an antidepressants for mild to moderate depression. The extract from this flower works by boosting serotonin levels.*

Q **I don't want to commit to years of therapy. Is there anything quicker?**

A *One that appeals to me is brief-focus therapy. Each session is treated as though it's your last although you may need four sessions. The therapist will ask you a miracle question. 'Imagine tonight there's a miracle and your problem goes away. How do you know the problem is gone?' Answering this question helps you clarify your problem-free future and should help you realise that your goals are within reach. Also, no matter what your problem is, it's not there all the time. For example, if you're miserable at work, there's usually the odd day or morning that's OK. Identifying what you did differently then tells you how you already cope with your problems. You can use this more consciously in future.*

25

Breathe easy

Think you've got sleep apnoea? Here's how to get diagnosed, what you can do yourself and what to expect in the hands of the experts.

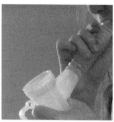

If lifestyle changes don't work, there's a vast array of medical devices built by teams of scientists designed to help you breathe easy again. Some of these – like wearing a huge mask every night – take a bit of getting used to, but it's a price worth paying for waking up refreshed.

So you think you might have sleep apnoea? See your doctor and bring along your regular partner, if you have one. Your doctor will ask about sleep and daytime sleepiness. He or she will look for abnormalities in your breathing passage such as a crooked nose or enlarged tonsils and may order blood tests to ensure your respiratory system and heart are normal.

You may then be referred to a sleep disorders clinic for overnight testing. Here you'll be hooked up to pads and electrodes and spend the night surrounded by

Here's an idea for you... **If you need to lose weight to help you breathe more easily at night, try one of the following psychological tricks to help you stick to your healthy eating plan. Stick an old picture of you when you were slimmer on the fridge to put you in the right frame of mind when you open it. Alternatively, a photo of you on the beach during your last holiday may make you more likely to grab the salad rather than the cheesecake.**

sophisticated machinery. While you're in the land of sleep, doctors will be checking your heart rhythm and blood oxygen levels. They'll also measure the effort to breathe by your chest and abdomen and check the airflow in front of your nose and mouth. By the morning they'll have found out how often you're waking up an hour, how long for and how low your blood oxygen levels are dropping when you stop breathing. Now, what to do about it?

HELPING YOURSELF

Your doctor will suggest some self-help remedies to begin with.

Lose weight. Fat deposits in your neck tissue can compress the airway and make it more likely to collapse. And a fat stomach can mean your breathing muscles work less efficiently, making it more difficult to breathe when you're asleep. Easier said than done, though. If you're seriously overweight, you've probably been on every diet going which, you probably already know by now, doesn't work. You lose weight quickly but will pile it on again just as fast. The only way to slim down for good is to lose no more than 2lb a week on a low-fat diet with plenty of fruit and vegetables. This demands willpower and a completely new approach to eating.

Give up smoking – this returns lung capacity to normal, making breathing easier. See your doctor about how to give up. And don't drink alcohol or take sleeping tablets, which both depress your breathing reflexes.

Try aromatherapy. Put a few drops of olbas, eucalyptus or peppermint oil in a diffuser at night – in one study essential oils reduced sleep apnoea in premature babies by 36%.

To get a better idea of whether you have sleep apnoea look at Idea 21, *Snores you can't ignore*.

Try another idea...

BRING ON THE EXPERTS

- Oral appliances – these are fitted by your dentist and bring your tongue and lower jaw forward, therefore widening the airway. Make sure you see a dentist who has regular contact with a sleep laboratory.
- Continuous positive airway pressure (CPAP) – currently the most successful treatment. When you're asleep you wear a mask over your nose, which blows air into your nose through a tube. This is connected to a small device which generates enough pressure to keep your airway from collapsing and open your breathing passage. It's a bit like putting air into a balloon – the walls simply spread apart. Although it's not going to make you feel sexy, it will probably improve your relationship as it usually gets rid of snoring and encourages regular breathing.
- Surgery. If the obstruction is caused by an abnormality in your nose or throat, then you may need surgery to fix it – particularly if it's caused by an obvious problem such as enlarged tonsils or adenoids. Nasal surgery opens nasal passages to correct a deviated septum. Jaw surgery is occasionally used to enlarge the lower and upper jaw, to make more room for the airway. Another operation involves getting rid of tissue from the back of the soft palate including the dangly bit at the back of the throat – or more technically the uvula. The success rate, however, is only about 50%.

'After two nights on the CPAP machine I felt like a 10-year-old who'd polished off a pot of coffee. I couldn't believe how refreshed I felt.'
GEORGE, sleep apnoea sufferer

Defining idea...

113

How did
it go?

Q   Does the CPAP machine work for everyone?

A   *It seems to work on about 70% of people with severe sleep apnoea. Some patients, however, have trouble getting used to the pressure in the nose or they develop symptoms of a blocked or runny nose.*

Q   I just can't face going to sleep wearing a mask with a tube dangling from it for the rest of my life. What do you suggest?

A   *If you wake up feeling awake and alert for the first time in years, it might be something worth suffering. It often takes a few weeks adjusting to the mask – make sure it's fitted properly, and that the pressure on the air compressor is set correctly for your needs. After a while, you won't be aware that you're even wearing it.*

Q   Isn't the noise of the CPAP machine just going to replace the sound of my husband's snoring?

A   *No – I can assure all long-suffering bed partners, the noise of the machine is similar to that of an air conditioner and far better than the noise of snoring. Some people even find the soft white noise of rushing air to be relaxing. If it does irritate you, try blocking the noise by putting the machine behind an item of furniture – a dresser, for instance.*

26

Sleep attack

Ask the average person about narcolepsy and they'll probably say they heard about it for the first time in *My Own Private Idaho* – a film where River Phoenix kept collapsing into a slumber at odd moments.

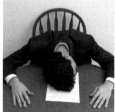

But, for the one in every 1,000 people who have narcolepsy, it's a potentially embarrassing and socially debilitating illness they have to live with every day.

Narcolepsy is a sleep disorder which makes you fall asleep at inappropriate times and places. It can begin at any age but once you've got it, you've got it for life. Sufferers are often very sleepy most of the time, but then have trouble falling asleep at night. As soon as they drop off, or start to wake up, they can have vivid, often frightening dreams and can also get sleep paralysis – making them unable to move temporarily.

The most well-known symptom is the sudden loss of muscle control triggered by laughter, surprise, fear or anger. It can be anything from a slight feeling of weakness and limp muscles to sudden total body collapse, during which the person looks asleep, but is in fact awake and alert. The attacks last from a few seconds up to 30 minutes.

Here's an idea for you... **Is there a pattern to your bouts of daytime tiredness? If so, don't fight the tiredness – plan naps around these times. Write down the times when you're normally overcome with fatigue, so during these danger times you can make sure you're in a nap-friendly environment. As well as drug therapy, many experts recommend two or three short naps during the day to help control sleepiness and maintain alertness.**

This happened to a women I was introduced to once. We were sitting in a pub eating dinner with a group of mutual friends and she was entertaining me with funny anecdotes about suddenly falling asleep in inappropriate situations. Then she laughed and promptly collapsed on the shoulder of her boyfriend, who was sitting next to her. Ten minutes later, she was chatting again.

It's very important to tell anyone you see regularly if you suffer from narcolepsy. People are incredibly understanding if they know the details. Your work colleagues may have noticed that you're not very alert at certain times of the day – and this would offer an explanation. A woman who talked about her condition to me was incredibly open – and was met by fascination in her condition rather than ridicule.

WHAT'S THE CAUSE?

Scientists have found a chemical in the brain that patients with narcolepsy seem to lack. Also, their rapid eye-movement (REM) sleep, which is when you're most likely to dream, seems to be all over the place. Normally, someone falls into REM sleep after about 90 minutes of sleep, but someone with narcolepsy can fall into REM sleep immediately so they often experience dreamlike imagery before the brain's asleep. REM episodes occur now and then in the day too – which is why people suffer hallucinations while they're awake.

Although symptoms of narcolepsy normally appear during adolescence, worryingly, it seems it's not being diagnosed. One study found that people had been suffering for about 15 years before it was recognised. If the only symptom is daytime sleepiness, sufferers are often treated for some other condition such as depression, which they may not have. This could make things worse – as some drugs used to treat depression can make the narcoleptic even sleepier. Children may be misdiagnosed with attention deficit disorder when they're actually just too tired to pay attention. As a result, they can give up on school.

Make the most of your napping time. Turn to IDEA 30, *Forty winks*, for the best places to nap, how to drop off and how long to nap for.

Try another idea...

TREATING NARCOLEPSY

It can't be cured, but with medication you'll be able to live a fairly normal life. The two main symptoms – daytime sleepiness and muscle weakness – are treated separately.

■ Modafinil – most commonly prescribed for excessive daytime sleepiness, it keeps you awake by working on the part of the brain that helps maintain alertness and has no side effects.

■ Ritalin – known as the medication prescribed to children with attention deficit hyperactivity disorder (ADHD) when it is used to calm them down and help them focus on their tasks. However, it helps to make people with narcolepsy more alert. But some people also suffer increased heart rate, rise in blood pressure and a jittery feeling.

'Having narcolepsy makes me feel like I've been given an anaesthetic.'

KERRY, narcolepsy sufferer

Defining idea...

- Tricyclic antidepressants – these have been used to help improve muscle control and REM symptoms.

Q Does narcolepsy affect fertility?

How did it go?

A *There's no evidence for this. The big issue is how to treat symptoms during pregnancy. You should probably stop using your medication just as you would most prescription and over-the-counter drugs. If alternative treatments such as daytime naps don't work, then you may have to take leave from work. You have to make sure you don't become deficient in iron and folic acid as this may cause restless legs syndrome.*

Q Can I drive?

A *Each country has different regulations – in some places you can't drive unless you're undergoing treatment. Even while on treatment, you mustn't drive late at night, when the medication may have worn off.*

Q How do I spot it in my teenage son?

A *He may start to sleep in and have to be dragged out of bed, even though he's gone to sleep at a normal time. He may fall asleep in school and his school performance may suddenly plummet. He'll always be sleepy. It'll be different from a normal sleep deprived teenager who becomes alert after a few good nights' sleep.*

27

No baby no cry

OK, so you didn't sort out your child's sleeping habits when she was a baby and now you're at your wits end. So here's the plan that stops your kids waking you up at night.

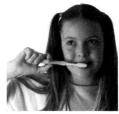

There are millions of parents out there who did the same when their children were babies and now run around every night dealing with their children's requests. At least you're prepared to do something about it now. A full night's sleep is within your grasp – I promise.

The key to every child's sleeping habits is the right bedtime routine which makes it easier for them to wind down to sleep. Once you've worked out a schedule, stick to it as well as keep bedtimes and waking times consistent seven days a week. So, for instance, you and your child may play quietly at 6, followed by bathtime at 6.30. Then you read to him for half an hour before putting him down to bed at 7.30. Having daytime routines such as regular meal and activity times also help anchor sleep times.

Here's an idea for you... **Try writing out your child's bedtime rituals like a script in order to make it consistent and put it up on the kitchen noticeboard where everyone can see it. They should be simple so that grandma or your babysitter can follow them if you're not around. A complicated ritual that requires a parent to be present makes it hard for a child to go back to sleep.**

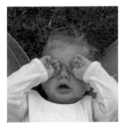

Bedtime routine established, you can now deal with those night-time wakings.

Most cases can be cured easily by controlled crying where you teach your child to go to sleep on her own. If you're really tough, you can probably solve it in two or three nights by letting her cry and not going to her at all. In theory, she'll cry for 20 or 30 minutes the first night (it'll probably seem like a couple of hours), 10 minutes the second night, not at all the third. You might find this approach too harsh – like I did – particularly if your child is between 6 and 19 months and is probably just suffering separation anxiety.

The solution for old softies, then, is to sit down by your baby's cot without turning on the light and keep murmuring something reassuring such as 'Don't worry, mummy (or daddy) is here. Go back to sleep' until she does. The idea is that you do less and less every night to comfort your baby until she's going to sleep on her own. If the first night you lightly stroke your baby, on the second night continue the soothing voice but don't stroke your child. Obviously, this takes a lot longer than the first method because it takes the child longer to realise she has to get herself to sleep.

If it's taking weeks and sleep deprivation is pushing you to the edge of insanity, you may want to try a compromise solution. On the first night, let your child cry for two minutes, then go in and reassure her briefly, tuck her in and leave; then let her cry for five, then ten, then fifteen and so on before going in to comfort her and leaving. This also usually works in a few nights, but may take up more of your night. So do it at a weekend when you and your partner can do shifts and make up for lost sleep the next day. Or recruit your brother or parents to do a night on duty.

When everyone is exhausted and you've already been up several times, it's tempting to take children into bed with you. And sometimes they just creep in without you knowing. If you've succumbed and now need to get the cuckoo back in its own nest, bear in mind that this may take a while. Explain that this bed is for adults and you would like your child to sleep in his or her bed. Be calm and ready to take your child back, perhaps many times, without getting cross. If they stay in their bed, but start crying, let them cry for a few minutes before going in to reassure them. Leave it a few minutes longer each time before going in.

Your child's bedroom environment is key for setting the scene for sleep. Take a look at IDEA 38, *Snoozy rooms*, which has tips on clearing the clutter and blocking out light.

Try another idea...

'Too many parents make life hard for their children by trying, too zealously, to make it easy for them.'

GOETHE

Defining idea...

Q   Is there anything I can do to make my child's bedroom more sleep friendly?

A   Children – like adults – depend on their environment for falling to sleep. Background noises, bedding, favourite toys and lighting can all affect your child's ability to fall asleep. A cool, dark, quiet room is best. Remove most toys, games, televisions, computers and radios if your child is having trouble falling asleep or is frequently up at night. These items can be powerful cues for wakefulness. One or two cuddly toys are fine, of course.

Q   Are there any over-the-counter remedies I can buy to help my child sleep?

A   I wouldn't recommend it. Medications become ineffective over time, and may make your child less alert during the day. They may also wear off during the night, and even cause night wakings. Some medications may also cause nightmares or other types of sleep disturbance.

28

Dreamworks

The average person will have over 1,800 dreams in one year – learn to control your dreams and they can help you tackle everyday problems. And this could mean you sleep better too.

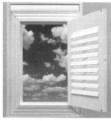

For most people dreams aren't particularly significant — they're simply something to laugh about with friends or colleagues over coffee. But with a bit of practice you can learn to use dreams to beat stress or even sort out problems.

How you interpret your dreams depends on who you are. Fans of Freud think dreams disguise people's repressed desires while Jungians think that by understanding the symbolic language of your dreams you can learn about all aspects of your personality. A therapist who uses dream therapy will encourage you to interpret your own dreams and help you work through your problems. And dream researchers can show you how to control your dreams and determine what happens in them – whether it's to stop a recurring nightmare or to help you sort out a tricky situation at work.

Here's an idea for you…

Try this experiment to see if you can influence your dreams. Before you go to bed imagine dreaming about (1) finding a light switch, (2) turning it on, then turning it off (3) turning on a light switch by willing it to happen and not touching the switch. Then see if any of these crop up in your dreams. In tests, 42% of people were able to incorporate these three tasks in their dream.

You can easily get into the habit of interpreting your dreams and, if you're lucky, you may even be able to control them without the help of a therapist. First off, make a habit of remembering your dreams. Keep a dream journal handy by your bed and record every dream you remember, no matter how fragmentary. Write them all down, not just the complete, coherent, or interesting ones – even if all you can recall is a face or a room. Remind yourself as you're falling asleep that you want to wake up fully from your dreams and remember them. This is similar to training yourself to wake up at a certain time in the morning.

After a week, look back at your dream journal and try to work out what it means – then take steps to address the concerns they may throw up. Think about the issues you have at work or in your relationship. Your dreams may point to problems you may not have thought of.

Learning to control your dreams – called lucid dreaming – is harder. This is when you realise you're dreaming, and then learn how to manipulate the dream. One man I know used the technique to dream about meeting a series of beautiful women who were magnetically attracted to him. However, it's probably more useful to use it to change the ending of recurrent dreams or nightmares or prepare for a forthcoming presentation or interview.

LEARN THE TECHNIQUE

A basic version is to think about the setting or topic of the dream before you go to sleep. If it's an interview, for instance, run through your mind the dialogue of the perfect interview. If you then dream about the interview going well, it will put you in the right frame of mind for the actual event. Or if you've got a question or dilemma that needs solving, think about this – and various outcomes – before bed. Your dream may clarify the problem – and a solution may pop into your head.

The advantage of a lucid dream is that you can see the effects of one outcome, then try another. Find out if you can lucid dream without guidance from a specialist – all you need to do is sit quietly for 10 minutes before going to bed, slow your breathing and keep telling yourself that you will become lucid when you're dreaming. Sounds simple, but it might be all you need to do. If you're trying to change the outcome of a recurrent dream then, when you're awake, write out the script of how you'd like it to end. Then read and visualise it for 10 minutes before you go to bed. Can't afford a massage? We'll if you want to wake up relaxed, imagine yourself having a massage in as much detail as possible. Think about how relaxed your shoulders and back will be. Then tell yourself you're going to become lucid and go to sleep and enjoy.

'A dream is a wish your heart makes, when you're fast asleep.'

Disney World advertisement

Defining idea...

For more ways to tackle stress, check out IDEA 22, *Say no to stress*. From putting your life in order to learning to say no, these strategies will stop stress in its tracks.

Try another idea...

How did it go?

Q   Does everyone dream?

A   *Although many people can't remember their dreams, research has shown that everyone dreams the same amount. Some people are just better at remembering them. And others wake more easily in REM sleep so recall more dreams than those who sleep more soundly.*

Q   If you're not controlling them, where do dreams come from?

A   *Your dreams are normally based on previous waking events, distorted in irrational ways. But by waking up out of a dream and immediately going over it, you can usually make some sense of it all.*

Q   But what do they mean?

A   *You need to ask yourself this after writing your dreams down. Being chased or running away could indicate that you're avoiding some problem or situation that needs to be taken care of. Falling could show that you're stepping into an unfamiliar situation and you're afraid of failure. The nude in public dream is very similar, and may show fear of embarrassment, or a lack of confidence in some area. Personal injury or losing body parts shows you're neglecting something. This may have to do with your body, such as diet or exercise, but could just as well indicate something you've neglected or forgotten elsewhere in your life – relationships or career, for instance.*

Q   How do you know if you're lucid dreaming?

A   *Learn to ask yourself if you're still dreaming when you're asleep. Then do something in the dream to prove that you're aware you're dreaming.*

29

Forget the lie in!

It's 5a.m. and one of your children comes into your bedroom wide awake, demanding to play a game of dominoes.

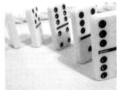

He hasn't had enough sleep and you know he'll be grumpy later on. And your body is screaming out for the extra two hours of sleep it needs.

If your children are waking up too early, you need to ask: are they getting up before they've had enough sleep or are they well rested and getting up earlier than you want them to? If your child is sleepy and wants to take a nap soon after rising – particularly if he's past the daytime napping stage – he's probably not getting enough sleep at night. Bear in mind that a toddler still needs around 12 hours sleep a night and a 3–5 year old needs around 11 hours.

IF YOUR CHILD'S SLEEPY ...

If your child is waking up before getting a full night's sleep, check to see whether something in his bedroom is rousing him or keeping him awake. If sunlight is

Here's an idea for you... **Start a star chart. Give your child a star every time she stays in her room until an agreed time – say, seven o'clock. After ten stars, allow her to choose a small treat from your local toy shop. If you're lucky, just getting the stars will be incentive enough.**

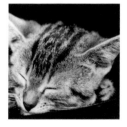

streaming in his window at the crack of dawn, for instance, hang curtains lined with blackout fabric or add a room-darkening shade or blind. The light is normally what tells the brain to wake up – but some children are more sensitive to it than others. If traffic or building work noise is the problem, keep your child's windows closed. A leaky nappy can be resolved by putting your toddler in super-absorbent night-time nappies. Cut down on night-time liquids, too. This will fill up a nappy and if he's potty trained, he may need the toilet at 5a.m. and be unable to get back to sleep.

If your child wakes early in the morning and you think he needs more rest, encourage him to go back to sleep. If your child is still in a cot and instead of rushing into his room the moment you hear a peep, wait ten or fifteen minutes – even if he's crying. He may just turn over and go back to sleep.

If your child needs you to help him go to sleep at night, chances are he'll need your help in the morning too. So you might have to go to his bed and reassure him, before returning to yours. Focus on teaching your child to go to sleep on his own when he goes to bed and he'll naturally get himself back to sleep at night or early in the morning if he wakes up.

IF HE'S HAD ENOUGH SLEEP …

If your toddler gets up raring to go at 5.30 or 6a.m, he's probably going to bed around 7 or 7.30p.m. Remember, your toddler can sleep only so much. For some children, a later bedtime will help. If your child's going to bed at 7, try tucking him in about ten minutes later every night until 7.30 or 8. But if you want a lie in, don't be tempted to put him to bed really late. Overtired children rarely sleep well and they'll probably get up the same time as they usually do anyway and just be grumpy the next day. Surprisingly, though, sometimes an earlier bedtime will help your toddler sleep later in the morning.

Encourage your child to play in their cot for a few minutes. Keeping a favourite toy or two in their cot can add valuable minutes to your sleep time. If you're child's older, try to get them to play with the toys in your bedroom until an agreed time – say, 7 o'clock. They don't need to be able to tell the time – just recognise when the big hand's at the 12 and the little hand's at the 7.

If your child also wakes up during the night, you'll probably be too tired to think properly during the day. For tips to stop night-time wakings, check out IDEA 14, Cry babies.

Try another idea…

'What is a home without children? Quiet.'

HENNY YOUNGMAN, comedian

Defining idea…

129

How did it go?

Q **My five-year-old son gets up between 5 and 5.30a.m. every morning – but refuses to go to bed until after 8.30. As a result he's often sleepy and grumpy in the day. What can I do?**

A *Is your son expending enough energy in the day? Children are a bit like dogs – they need an hour's run every day. Research has shown that this is the key to good night's sleep in children. So give your son lots of exercise and fresh air during the day plus plenty of relaxing and unwinding at night. And make sure he has a regular bedtime: bath, then quiet time, books and bed at the same time every evening.*

Q **My daughter wakes up early claiming she's hungry – although I know she hasn't had enough sleep. So I'm downstairs preparing breakfast at 5.30 every morning. How can I break the habit?**

A *By feeding your daughter as soon as she wakes up, you've trained her tummy to wake at daybreak. Instead delay it until 8 o'clock – using a ten minutes a day approach until you have breakfast time where you want it. If she's really hungry give her a light snack like a cracker or rice cake. The idea is that she'll gradually wake up later too.*

Q **If I want my daughter to wake up later, should I stop her afternoon nap?**

A *Not if she needs it and won't be able to last until bedtime. Just make sure it's not after 4. Although she may still go to bed at her usual bedtime, she's more likely to wake up early.*

30

Forty winks

If you find yourself feeling sleepy after lunch, perhaps a siesta is what you need, but does the power nap really work?

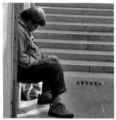

Whether you're preparing for an important meeting or tidying up at home, on some afternoons it's virtually impossible to fight the urge to sleep. Should you give in and enjoy a bit of shut-eye or will it make it even more difficult to get to sleep at night?

We're designed for two sleeps a day – the main one at night and a nap in the afternoon. A drop in temperature makes us feel sleepy between 2 and 4p.m. If you're getting enough sleep at night, you'll probably be OK – a handful of nuts may be all you need to pep you up.

If you're sleep deprived, though, you could be under par all afternoon. Suddenly you need to stretch, move about, yawn or sigh. You might find it harder to concentrate and your mind will start wandering. You could even start making typing errors and find it more difficult to find the right word when you're speaking.

Here's an idea for you... **To discover how naps affect your energy level and the quality of your night-time sleep, do an experiment. Take a daily nap for a week. The next week, don't nap. Every morning, rank your sleep quality on a 10-point scale. Every evening, rate your day on a similar scale. After two weeks, judge whether naps work for you.**

According to fans of napping, if you just grab a coffee and push on, you're denying your body its natural restorative period. But a 15- to 20-minute nap, they say, can restore alertness and memory and relieve stress and fatigue. You're also less likely to fall asleep in front of the TV later on, then be unable to drop off at bedtime.

In reality, though, it's often difficult to nap. If you're looking after children, you can't leave them unsupervised for 20 minutes and although some companies are beginning to allow napping – particularly those that rely on shift workers – most don't. But even if you don't actually fall asleep, 20 minutes of quiet time may give you the boost you need.

NICE NAPPING

- Find somewhere quiet.
- If you're working in an office, switch your phone to voicemail and either sit at your desk or find an empty room. Ideally you'd hang a sign on your door saying 'Do not disturb' and get your secretary to wake you 20 minutes later. But we're not all company directors.
- Loosen your clothing and take off your shoes. Lie down on a sofa, stretch out on the floor or if that's not possible sit comfortably on a chair, placing your head in your folded arms on your desk.

- Close your eyes – ideally, put on an eye mask.
- Try not to think about work or all the things you have to do. Focus on what you love doing in your spare time. If you like golf, you might mentally play a round of golf on your regular course. Maybe drift back to a favourite holiday, or listen to some calming music.
- Just rest at first – if your brain needs a rest as well, you'll soon fall asleep.
- Set the alarm to go off in twenty minutes' time, in case you do fall asleep. Don't sleep for more than 30 minutes – you'll wake up groggier and foggier.
- When you wake up lie still for a minute or two – then stretch and breathe deeply and take a drink of water or a light snack to get your system going again.
- Then, return to work, starting with simple chores such as opening letters or organising the work you have to do. Within just a few minutes you should feel sparky again.

'No day is so bad it can't be fixed with a nap.'
CARRIE SNOW, comedian

Defining idea...

NAPPING WITH A BABY

If you've got a young baby who wakes up constantly at night taking short naps might well help you get through the day until your baby begins to follow a more consistent sleep schedule (usually around three or four months). If you're at home with your baby, nap when she does. If you work outside your home, try flexible working or reserve blocks of time to nap during your working day if that's possible. However, if you

Having trouble dropping off? Try the visualisation techniques in IDEA 32, *Mind power*, or find out how music can help you tune out in IDEA 41, *Music to my ears*.

Try another idea...

have problems falling asleep at bedtime, or find you are still waking in the night even though your baby is sleeping through, give up daytime naps. Don't make up for a restless night by sleeping late or going to bed earlier than usual, either. This can turn a short-term sleep problem into a long-term sleep disturbance. If you begin to feel drowsy during the day, stay active by cleaning the house, exercising or visiting a friend.

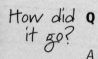

How did it go?

Q   Can naps make up for lack of sleep?

A   *If you're not getting enough sleep, napping may help in the short term, but it's not the cure for insomnia. In fact, it could make sleeping at night more difficult. You need to deal with the cause of your insomnia. If you don't have insomnia, but you regularly have to go to bed later than you want to, a daytime nap might give you the boost you need.*

Q   There's no chance of a nap in the day where I work. What do you suggest?

A   *If napping is not possible, gaze out of a window and daydream for 5–10 minutes or stretch, walk around and maybe massage your neck. If you can't even take a rest, the next best thing is to change tasks and the pace at which you are working. So organise your things to do for tomorrow, doodle on a note pad, let voicemail take your calls or do filing, tidy your desk and clear out clutter.*

31

Pill popping

The lowdown on sleeping pills. Is it really a short cut to good sleep?

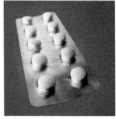

We've come a long way since the 1960s and 1970s when very strong, incredibly addictive barbiturates were routinely prescribed for insomnia, and stars like Marilyn Monroe and Jimi Hendrix were dying from overdoses of these powerful pills.

Newer pills are gentler and more effective – but are they the best way to solve your sleeping problems?

Experts can't make up their mind about them. Some think they're a good short-term measure for insomnia, others think they're not tackling the cause and you risk becoming dependent on them. Like with caffeine or nicotine, you can get physically – as well as psychologically – addicted. You take them every day and get a good night's sleep, but as soon as you stop taking them the sleeplessness returns. Why? You haven't dealt with what's causing your insomnia and you still can't go to sleep on your own.

Here's an idea for you...

Take this checklist to your doctor if you're considering prescription sleeping pills.

- To ensure you get the right pill for you, describe your problem precisely – whether you can't go to sleep or you wake up frequently, whether you're stressed or depressed, for instance.
- Once your doctor has chosen the sleeping pill, ask them to read out the description in their medical bible MIMS. What is it designed to do, how does it work, what are the possible side effects, how long is it likely to be effective?
- Ask what dosages are available. Insist on the lowest dose pack. You don't want to get hooked on a higher dose and at some time you will need to wean yourself off.

Most doctors prefer giving out antidepressants which they think of as a lower-risk option to help tackle the cause of insomnia.

The sleeping pills your doctor will prescribe work by depressing your brain activity and slowing down brainwaves. They also make you sleep by relieving anxiety and relaxing your muscles. The difference betwcen the various brands is usually the time it takes for the effects to wear off – that is the time it takes the body to break them down and get them out of your system. This can be anything from a few hours to days – the longer they hang around, the more likely you are to feel drowsy or suffer other side effects.

Also, the longer you use sleeping pills, the more your brain gets used to them and the less effective they are. After four to six weeks your sleeping pill will probably be as useful as an extra strong mint. Of course, the answer is not to increase your dose. You need to stop taking them.

Another thing to bear in mind is that sleeping pills don't necessarily give you more sleep – they often give you less, in fact. This is because most new-generation sleeping pills are best at knocking you out and putting you to sleep. They don't tend to last more than four hours so you could still wake up in the night or wake up too early. Sleeping pills increase stage 2, or light sleep, but lessen deep sleep and REM sleep (which is why often you recall dreams much less on sleeping pills). So ironically the quality of your sleep may suffer, too.

There are two types of sleeping pill most commonly prescribed – benzodiazepines such as temazepam, flurazepam and lorazepam which help relax muscles and imidazopyridines and cyclopyrrolones such as zolpidem, salepon and zoplicone which also relax the muscles. They don't last as long as the first type but they're less addictive and you're less likely to feel drowsy in the day. Different sleeping pills have slightly different effects – you may have to try a few before you find one that suits you.

Before using sleeping pills, try more than simply one other idea – give all the ideas a go. Start with sorting out your sleep routine in IDEA 7, *Back to basics*, reducing your stress levels in IDEA 22, *Say no to stress*, and making sure your bedroom is giving the right sleep signals in IDEA 38, *Snoozy rooms*.

Try another idea…

'Reality is just a crutch for people who can't cope with drugs.'

ROBIN WILLIAMS

Defining idea…

137

Q What are the side effects?

A *You probably won't get any if you only use them occasionally – just a little feeling of morning-after euphoria perhaps. But over a long period of time, it can worsen your memory and concentration and make you less alert. Some people feel like they're in a daze. Others have side effects such as headaches, nausea or nightmares. People who are or have been dependent on sleeping pills have a much harder job curing their insomnia in the long run. You would need expert help and support to wean yourself off.*

Q Is there any research to support taking sleeping tablets?

A *A Canadian study found that taking sleeping pills worked in the short-term, but only changing their behaviour was effective over a long period. Strategies that worked best include not using your bed for activities such as eating or reading – only sleeping and sex; getting out of bed and going to another room if you can't fall asleep within 15 to 20 minutes of going to bed; and getting up at the same time in the morning each day, regardless of how much sleep you've had.*

Q How do you wean yourself off sleeping pills?

A *You do it gradually by reducing the dose. Sometimes this will mean cutting your pill in half, then a quarter and so on. You may then use an over-the-counter sleeping pill every now and again. These contain antihistamines – usually found in cold and allergy remedies – which have sedative effects. They don't put you to sleep, but make you drowsy so you can fall asleep faster. Like sleeping tablets, you get used to them so they'll only work for a few weeks.*

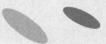

32

Mind power

Forget expensive gadgets and sleeping pills to send you into a slumber – use your brain to help you switch off.

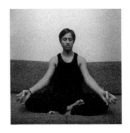

You know how easy it is for your thoughts to spiral out of control. Well, with a bit of direction, you can rein in your thoughts and think yourself sleepy. Here's how.

First off, you probably need to become more positive about sleep – particularly if you've got to the stage that you dread going to bed, convinced that you're never going to get a good night's sleep again. This mindset will make your insomnia worse. Try to replace any negative thoughts with positive ones – not unconvincing ones that you don't really believe like 'I'm going to have the best night's sleep I've ever had tonight.' Instead go for 'As long as I get some sleep and relax my body, I'll be fine.' So every time you catch yourself with a negative thought about sleep, give it a more positive spin. The idea behind positive affirmations is that if you say them enough, you'll believe them. Writing them down may speed up this process. So if you're thinking 'I can't get enough sleep', the positive spin could be 'I don't need as much sleep as I think. I can function very well on less.'

Don't want to visualise a peaceful or relaxing scene? Why not think of something or somewhere that you've always found really boring? It could be listening to a particular teacher who was so boring that he or she almost always put you to sleep. Perhaps it's some friend who can't stop talking. Maybe it's a particularly boring part of your work, like the filing, or simply sitting on the bus on the way to work. Whatever it is, visualise it. And recapture that bored, tired, heavy, sleepy feeling that you always experience. Let that feeling spread through your mind and all through your body until you're overcome with tiredness.

Another trick is to associate your bedroom with relaxing. Good sleepers cultivate strong mental associations of physical relaxation, mental calm and good sleep with their bedtime, their bed and bedroom, and their bedtime rituals like tooth brushing and setting the alarm clock. You can learn to become a good sleeper by making these same associations. Practising muscle relaxation while you're brushing your teeth, deep breathing while you're putting on your pyjamas. And imagine your bed is a huge white fluffy cloud and that all your worries disappear the moment you step into it.

Take this visualisation further when you're in bed by conjouring up an image of something relaxing. Just lie there with your eyes closed and imagine you're in your favourite, most peaceful place. It may be on a sunny beach, swinging in a hammock in the mountains or all alone in a cave in the Himalayas.

Wherever it is, try to experience it in your head – see your surroundings, hear the peaceful sounds, smell the fragrance of the flowers, and feel the warmth of the sun. Just relax and enjoy it – and drift off to sleep. Once you've found a place that's especially peaceful and effective, you'll find that the more you use it, the more you can count on it to help you relax and get to sleep.

'I really can't be expected to drop everything and start counting sheep at my age. I hate sheep.'

DOROTHY PARKER

Defining idea...

If you're finding it hard to think of anything relaxing apart from a beach, which is a bit of a cliché, why not imagine you're standing under a waterfall – recent research says the most relaxing way to drop off is being near a waterfall. A stream of water (warm or cool) gently cascades over your head, running downwards over the outside of your body, taking with it tensions and negative thoughts, which soak into the ground. Repeat three times. Next imagine the water is entering the crown of your head, and running through your body. Use your imagination to visualise its force cleansing your organs, joints, digestive tract and so on. The idea is that the water will drain the negative thoughts and toxins out of your body through the soles of your feet and down into the earth.

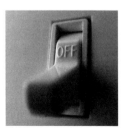

If you want to take your mind off your worries and your partner's lying next to you, why not have sex? Find out more about the world's most enjoyable insomnia cure in IDEA 36, *Sexual healing*.

Try another idea...

How did it go?

Q **Why does thinking positively help you sleep?**

A *Negative thoughts and emotions release stress chemicals that stop the production of your sleep hormones and release ones that keep you awake. Positive thoughts, however, relax you and get you in the mood for sleep.*

Q **Worries swim around my head and stop me going to sleep, but thinking about something beautiful or boring doesn't seem to help. Any suggestions?**

A *Visualise putting your worries away last thing at night. You could, for instance, put them in a file, close the file firmly and file them away into a filing cabinet. Lock the cabinet and walk away. Or you could put your worries in a hot air balloon. Visualise the colour of the balloon and set it in breathtaking scenery with blue skies and fluffy white clouds. Undo the ties and let your cares float away. Another idea is to turn your worries into little creatures that you put away in a box. Think about the colour of the box and how big it is. Shut the box tight and put it somewhere safe for the morning.*

Q **I sometimes wake in the night and start worrying. How can I get back to sleep?**

A *You can't solve problems in the middle of the night. Train yourself to say 'It'll sort itself out' or 'I can't do anything about it now', or 'I'll see things more clearly tomorrow'. You're not denying the problem, but you want to banish those kinds of thoughts from the bed.*

33

Food for thought

What and when you eat affects how you sleep – so read on for the dinners to make you doze.

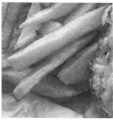

Late night pizzas, take-away curries, chips ... If this is a list of what you've enjoyed for your evening meals over the last week, it's not surprising you've been sleeping badly.

Eating healthily and regularly is one of the best ways to keep your energy levels high, stopping you dropping off inappropriately in the day and ensuring your body releases all the hormones you need to send you off to sleep at night. The most effective sleep diet is to eat little and often rather than one or two big meals, which keeps your metabolic rate steady. This is particularly key for your evening meal – your metabolic rate and temperature will shoot up after a big meal when they should be dropping to prepare for sleep. Your digestive system has to work harder too. While you may fall asleep faster, all the intestinal work required to digest a big meal is likely to cause frequent waking and a poorer quality of sleep. Your sleep can also be affected by foods which take a long time to digest – high fat and high pro-

Write down what and when you eat and drink in your sleep diary for a week and see if there's any link between your diet and how well you sleep. You can then start by avoiding any food that's causing problems.

tein foods take twice as long as carbohydrate to metabolise. So if you were tossing and turning after last night's chicken tikka massala, you know why.

CALMING FOODS

One of the keys to a restful night's sleep is to get your brain calmed rather than revved up. So you need to avoid foods that perk you up and opt for ones that encourage restful sleep. Steer clear of foods containing the amino acid tyrosine – found in bacon, cured meat, strong cheese (mild ones are fine) and chocolate – which stimulate the brain. Instead go for those containing tryptophan – an amino acid that your body uses to make serotonin, which it then turns into sleep-inducing melatonin. Your body doesn't make tryptophan, so the only way you can get it is by eating foods that contain it like cottage cheese, milk, chicken, turkey, rice, eggs, beans, spinach and seafood. To get the full snoozy effect, however, you need to eat these foods with carbohydrates such as pasta or potatoes. After eating carbs, your body releases insulin, which helps clear the bloodstream of other amino acids that compete with tryptophan. This means more tryptophan gets to the brain – and more of those lovely sleep hormones get made. Clever, eh?

Although you need a balance of vitamins to keep your sleep functions ticking along, there are a few key ones. Vitamin B6, for instance, triggers the pineal gland in the brain to secrete more melatonin. They're in wholegrains, bananas, dried apricots and potatoes. Vitamin B3, found in red meat, chicken, oily fish and mushrooms, has been shown to improve REM sleep and decrease waking time in the night. And boosting levels of magnesium (in avocados, green leafy veg and nuts) and calcium (dairy products, broccoli, almonds) reduces the time it takes to get to sleep and the amount of times you wake up at night.

Nearly bedtime and still peckish? Go to IDEA 34, *Sleepy snacks* for some slumber-inducing bites.

Try another idea…

DINNERS THAT HELP YOU DROP OFF

Meals that are high in carbohydrates and low to medium in protein will help you relax in the evening and set you up for a good night's sleep. Good ones to try are:

- Baked potato with cottage cheese and tuna salad
- Chicken breast, potatoes and green beans
- Pasta with spinach and pinenuts
- Wholewheat spaghetti with bean, tofu or meat sauce
- Salmon fillet and green salad with yoghurt dressing
- Pasta with tomatoes and lentils
- Tuna steak with boiled potatoes and spinach
- Avocado pasta salad
- Scrambled eggs on wholemeal toast and cheese
- Tofu stir-fry
- Hummus with wholewheat pita bread
- Seafood pasta
- Chicken stir-fry with pasta and vegetables
- Tuna salad sandwich
- Tuna salad sprinkled with sesame seeds (rich in tryptophan), and wholewheat crackers

'A light supper, a good night's sleep, and a fine morning have often made a hero of the same man who by indigestion, a restless night, and a rainy morning, would have proved a coward.'

LORD CHESTERFIELD

Defining idea…

145

How did it go?

Q **You talk about eating to sleep. But what about eating to keep me awake in the day too?**

A *You need to keep eating small amounts, preferably every three or four hours. If you starve yourself, you'll have no energy – and you won't feel sleepy later on either. But avoid fatty or sugary snacks like crisps, biscuits or chocolate – the blood sugar boost of these foods will temporarily pep you up – but an hour later you'll feel even worse. Good snacks to have mid morning, mid afternoon and evening include: a small handful of dried fruit and nuts, chopped apple or orange and low-fat yoghurt or a small portion of low-fat cottage cheese with pineapple. A pick-me-up lunch should be heavier on protein than carbohydrates, since protein-rich foods contain the stimulating amino acid tyrosine. Try a chicken or tuna salad. And keep drinking water – you'll feel tired if you get dehydrated.*

Q **I eat a lot of garlic. Could it be affecting my sleep?**

A *Yes, some people find that highly seasoned foods such as garlic, spices and hot peppers interfere with sleep, especially if you suffer from heartburn. And foods containing the additive monosodium glutamate, found in many processed foods and take-aways, can cause headaches, heartburn and digestive problems as well as disrupt your sleep.*

Q **Does this mean I can't have pizza ever again?**

A *No of course not – just not every night. As well as disrupting your sleep, a daily diet of pizzas and other convenience food would make most people overweight which can trigger other sleep problems like snoring and sleep apnoea.*

146

34

Sleepy snacks

It's nearly time to hit the hay and you're not tired yet. Why not have a bedtime bite to kickstart those snooze hormones?

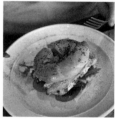

Many foods contain natural sedatives that stimulate the brain to produce calming chemicals which make you feel drowsy. Eat the wrong thing, though, and you could find yourself more awake than you were before.

A bedtime snack can not only help you drop off, it can stop you waking up in the middle of the night with a rumbling tummy. If you fall asleep easily but awaken several hours later, it may be due to low blood sugar – and a light bite before bed could nip that in the bud. You need to eat a high carbohydrate snack which has some fat just before you go to sleep. A banana works well as it digests slowly and helps your body release sleep hormones later in the night.

To help you go to sleep in the first place, you need something that's high in complex carbohydrates, with a small amount of protein which contains just enough tryptophan to relax the brain. A bit of calcium on top of this works a treat – it helps the brain use the tryptophan to make the sleep hormone melatonin. In fact the

Here's an
idea for
you... **Instead of hot milk, make this oaty alternative. Soak a level tablespoon of oatmeal in milk for an hour or so in a small saucepan. Add a large glass of milk and bring to the boil gently, stirring all the time until it has slightly thickened. Pour it back into a glass, then add a spoonful of honey and plenty of grated nutmeg. You'll soon feel your eyelids get heavier and heavier ...**

age-old sleep aid, a bowl of porridge, is probably the best sleep-inducing food of all as it contains, complex carbohydrates, calcium and tryptophan. Some 40 minutes later, your levels of melatonin will rise – setting you up for a deep, restorative sleep.

Avoid all-carbohydrate snacks, especially those high in junk sugars like biscuits – they're less likely to help you sleep. You'll miss out on the sleep-inducing effects of tryptophan, and you may set off the roller-coaster effect of plummeting blood sugar followed by the release of stress hormones that will keep you awake.

And yes, that old wives' tale about cheese before bed giving you nightmares is true. Cheese – particularly mature ones – contains the amino acid tyramine, which triggers the release of adrenaline. This stimulates your brain and can trigger vivid dreams as well as nightmares. The fat in cheese can also give you bad dreams – fatty food is more difficult to digest particularly when you're asleep as your digestive system automatically slows down. So while an army of enzymes tries to break down the fat, your sleep is being disrupted and you're dreaming of being chased by a giant piece of Brie.

RECIPES FOR SLEEP ...

Try one of these healthy snacks about 40 minutes before you settle down under your duvet. This gives them enough time to perform their magic ...

- Honey with oatcakes
- Wholemeal toast with cottage cheese and pineapple
- Yoghurt and strawberries (yoghurt contains natural sleep-inducing substances called casomorphins)
- 3 sticks of celery and low-fat fromage frais (celery contains a substance called 3-n-butyl phthalide, which acts as a gentle sedative)
- Banana slices and fromage frais
- Bagel with low-fat cream cheese and chopped dates
- Crackers and hummus
- Wholegrain cereal with milk
- Hazelnuts and tofu
- Peanut butter sandwich and ground sesame seeds – both of which contain tryptophan
- A few slices of lettuce – not a very exciting snack, but full of natural sedatives

If you're still not sleepy, wind down with some simple stretches from IDEA 42, *Say yes to yoga*, or try a meditation technique from IDEA 43, *Ommmm ...*

Try another idea...

If you fancy a snoozy bedtime drink to accompany your snack, then nothing beats a mug of warm milk and honey. But you can also try a milkshake made with skimmed milk, strawberries and low fat frozen yoghurt or a milkshake using soya milk (soya contains tryptophan). Alternatively, make your own herbal infusion from limeflower, lemon balm and lavender adding half a teaspoon of each to a mug of hot water. Cover (to prevent the plant oils evaporating), infuse for five minutes then sweeten with honey to taste.

'My favourite bedtime snack is Bran Flakes topped with maple and pecan muesli. Alternatively a Kit Kat – but they're strictly for midnight feasts only!'
ANNA FOSTER, morning breakfast radio show host

Defining idea...

149

How did
it go?

Q   Is it worth having a snack even if you've had a late dinner?

A   *Tryptophan works best on an empty stomach so your snack will have maxi-mum impact only if you've had dinner two or three hours earlier.*

Q   What about a tipple before bedtime?

A   *Under no circumstances drink alcohol before bed. It blocks tryptophan so all the good effects of those sleepy snacks will go to waste.*

Q   Can you take these sleep hormones as supplements?

A   *Although they're not a substitute for a good diet and sound nutrition, some experts still think they're a good way of boosting various sleep-promoting substances. There are plenty of supplements available but in some coun-tries they're only available on prescription, not over the counter. As there have been no published trials it's difficult to vouch for their effectiveness too. All positive results are anecdotal. The supplement 5-HTP (5-hydroxy-tryptophan) converts to serotonin in your body and is extracted from the seeds of a West African plant. It's used for insomnia that's related to anxiety. L-tryptophan is the pill form of tryptophan and there have been reports of it raising levels of sleep-inducing melatonin by 300% in only ten minutes. It should only be seen as a short-term measure, though. And melatonin supplements, which are often taken for jet lag, can help insom-nia – but they don't have the mood-boosting benefits of the other two.*

35

Fit for sleep

You already know that keeping fit makes you look better, feel better and live longer – but did you know it can sort out your sleep problems too?

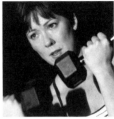

Regular exercise can actually help you drop off more quickly and sleep more soundly. You've got no excuses now — grab your trainers and get moving.

If you're a poor sleeper, your metabolism, heart rate and body temperature all shoot up during sleep. When you exercise, however, your metabolism goes up initially but after a few hours, your body temperature and metabolism drop more than if you hadn't worked out – so you're less likely to wake up in the night. Studies have shown you'll also get more deep sleep. And exercise not only cuts your stress – a big cause of insomnia – a chemical released when you're doing aerobic exercise protects you from the harmful effects of stress.

You need to do at least three hours a week, though, to make a difference. You don't need to do it all at once – ten minutes three times a day works just as well as one

Here's an idea for you... **Start an exercise diary. Note down every activity you do every day and how long you did it for – everything from walking to the bus stop to those star jumps you did while watching *Celebrity Big Brother* on TV. Then note how well you slept that night. Work out if any particular activity is helping you sleep. Once you've reached your weekly three-hour aerobic target, give yourself a reward.**

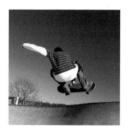

half-hour session. Although aerobic exercise – anything that gets your heart pumping faster – works best, lifting weights and stretching can also help your sleep.

The important thing is when to exercise. The ideal time is late afternoon or evening – if you do a strenuous workout too close to bedtime your temperature may be still be too high for sleep. You need to wait for your body to cool down – about three to four hours – as a fall in temperature is an important trigger for sleep.

FIT EXERCISE INTO YOUR LIFE

■ Do something you enjoy – you'll only give up otherwise. If you can't motivate yourself to go running or work out in a gym, think seriously about what will keep your interest. If you're competitive, try team sports. If you're sociable, do a dance class or join a hiking club. If you need a challenge, try wall climbing or a martial art where you're learning a skill as well as getting fit.

- Set a goal – whether it's to run around the park without collapsing in a heap gasping for breath or, if you're doing yoga, to be able to touch your toes for the first time in your life. And as soon as you've reached your goal, set another.
- Change your activities regularly. Boredom is one of the main reasons people stop exercising. Do an activity you've never done before like t'ai chi or a spinning class. Not for you? Try something else.
- If you work regular hours, walk or cycle part or all of the way to work. Start with just once a week, then progress to two to three times a week.
- Make life a bit difficult for yourself. During your lunch hour, find a sandwich shop 15 minutes' walk away rather than the one next to your office – and walk briskly. Forget about the car for short journeys – like popping to the shops to get a pint of milk or returning a video. And it goes without saying that you take the stairs at work and use steps not lifts or escalators in department stores.
- Keep giving up on your exercise video? Get a fan. Research has found that getting too hot may be putting off exercisers – a cool breeze will make you more alert and willing to hang on to the end.

If you're slow to get going in the morning, do the moves in IDEA 49, *Wake-up stretches* – guaranteed to clear your head and lift your spirits.

Try another idea...

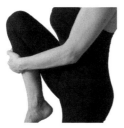

'Whenever I feel like exercising, I lie down until the feeling passes.'
ROBERT MAYNARD HUTCHINS,
education reformer

Defining idea...

How did it go?

Q **I live right next to a park so I try to go running. I don't seem to be able to run for more than 10 minutes without getting bored. So I give up. Any tips?**

A *First, get some headphones. Listening to fast beat music has been shown to make people exercise harder and for longer. Secondly, be patient. It takes 21 sessions to make exercise a habit – so if you're running three times a week, it'll take about 7 weeks before your body expects to go for a run. After that, it'll be much easier. I promise.*

Q **I look after my children full time so how can I possibly fit in any exercise?**

A *Well, if your children are young, they're probably keeping you pretty active anyway. If not, simply incorporate some of your exercise into your daily routine. Run up and down the stairs three times, do a mini circuit in your home including sit-ups, jogging on the spot, press-ups and other strengthening exercises. Do a swap with another parent – they look after your kids while you go for a run and vice versa. At the weekend, try to organise family fitness events – go for a bike ride or a long walk.*

Q **I work long, irregular hours – how can I fit in exercise?**

A *Invest in a fitness video and use it at least once a week. Buy a skipping rope – ten minutes of vigorous skipping in your living room will leave you exhausted. Jog up and down during commercial breaks on TV. Do at least two 15-minute walks a day – remember that cumulative exercise is just as important as intense bouts. Do ten minutes of vigorous cleaning twice a day. Spend an hour working in the garden at the weekend. Get the idea?*

36

Sexual healing

Why even consider sleeping tablets if a few moments of passion with your partner can do the trick?

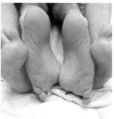

Regular sex not only does wonders for your relationship, it also helps you unwind from the day's stresses and triggers some important sleep-inducing hormones. Now where did you put that thong ...?

After a hectic day when the dog was sick, your computer broke down, you had an argument with your boss and, to cap it all, you got a parking ticket, the only thing you can think of is the large glass of red wine waiting for you when you get home. What you should be thinking about though is an evening of passion – guaranteed to blast your stress and send you to sleep relaxed.

If you feel you just don't have time for sex, you're not alone. The hectic pace of 21st-century life, soaring stress levels and long working hours have taken their toll on people's sex lives. In one survey, less than a third of women have the average amount of sex – at least twice a week – and 43% suffer from low libido.

Here's an idea for you... **Improve your orgasms – perform kegal exercises. By exercising the muscles you use to control your urine flow you can improve your control and your sensation when you have sex. Both men and women can do this. Just tense then relax these muscles slowly. Start by doing 10, but build up to 100 a day (don't worry – no one will know you're doing them).**

When you have an orgasm, your body releases five times the normal level of the cuddle hormone oxytocin, which calms you down for sleep. Orgasms also produce a rush of endorphins which lift your spirits. One study even found that a shot of semen boosts the mood of women with depression – many of whom suffer sleep problems. It seems that the vagina absorbs all the nutrients found in semen – zinc, calcium, potassium, fructose and various proteins – which makes its way into the bloodstream a few hours later.

And if headaches are preventing you from getting to sleep, sex may be just what the doctor ordered. Most headaches are tension headaches and muscle tension is usually found in your head, shoulders, neck or back. After you've had sex, the feelgood endorphins released act like a mild painkiller.

There's nothing like a runny nose to disrupt your sleep either. Sex, however, can boost your immune system by triggering the release of antibodies into the mucosal immune system in the mouth, lungs and gastrointestinal tract, blocking the passage of viruses and bacteria into the bloodstream.

Most important, good sex life brings you closer to your partner because of the intimacy you share. And if you're happy with your partner, it's one thing less to worry about when you're trying to get to sleep. And it seems the more of it you get, the better – one study found that people who have more sex feel happier in their relationships and at work and have learned how to handle stress better.

REV UP YOUR SEX LIFE

- Flirt with each other – over breakfast, while you're brushing your teeth, in the queue at the post office, everywhere.
- Throw your TV out of the bedroom – watching TV in bed hypnotises you into wanting to sleep and kills off your sex life.
- Don't skip the kissing. It makes sex last longer, strengthens affection and arousal.
- Give each other a massage. Using oil, give each other a 10-minute massage. Don't spoil it by talking about mortgage payments, though. Or for something a bit naughtier, try a body-to-body massage – man on his front, woman on top. Rub your body up and down his.
- Eat a banana in bed. A rich source of vitamin B they enhance sex and orgasm by promoting the flow of blood to your sex organs.
- Go to bed naked – there's nothing like baggy jogging pants and a holey T-shirt to put you off sex. Leave a T-shirt by the bed for if you get cold later.
- Talk to each other – it's the key to good sex and a lively libido – and before you say you're too busy, it doesn't take much time. Set aside a time each day – between 9 and 9.30p.m. for instance, when you don't watch TV, you actually catch up and talk. Go out together once a week – and bring back that first date feeling

Not sure your massage skills are up to scratch? For a detailed step-by-step on how to perform the perfect aromatherapy massage, check out IDEA 46, *It makes scents*.

Try another idea…

'When I'm good I'm very, very good but when I'm bad I'm better.'

MAE WEST

Defining idea…

157

by sometimes arranging to meet at the restaurant separately. And get away for weekends – if you have children, get grandma or auntie to look after them. By setting aside time on a weekend away or a romantic night in, you're telling each other you're important – and are learning to enjoy each other's company again. Then you can start talking about sex. Ask each other what you enjoy doing, whether you want to try something different – new positions perhaps? Don't make it serious – have fun with it.

How did it go?

Q   Why does my husband always go to sleep seconds after sex while it takes me about half an hour?

A   Men are often more affected by the intense wave of calm and relaxation after they orgasm and are often struck by an incredibly strong urge to go to sleep. This is particularly true if they're tired anyway and are just being kept up by stressful thoughts. The hormones released during an orgasm seems to drug them temporarily before their thoughts can return.

Q   My husband always complains that I fall asleep as soon as we get into bed. What can I do?

A   That's an easy one. Go to bed before you're tired. And don't go to bed stressed – take time out to relax. Libido, like our appetite for food, is affected by many things such as stress and anxiety. Why not enjoy a pre-bed bath – preferably together.

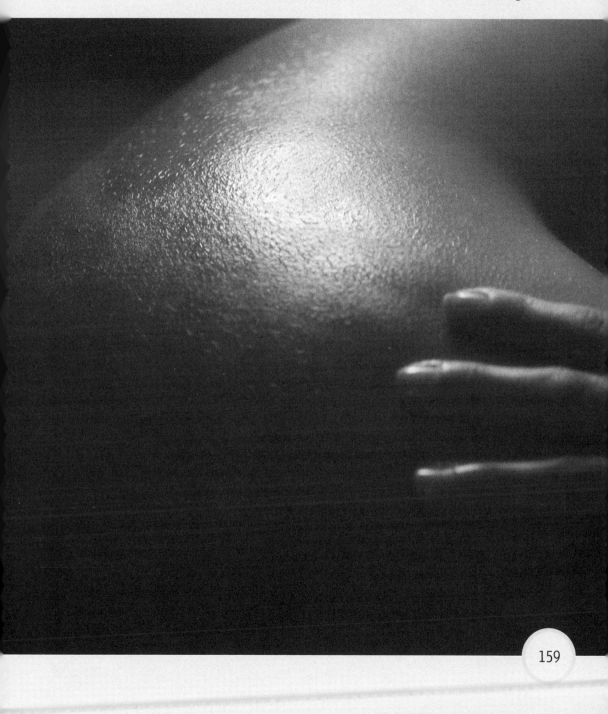

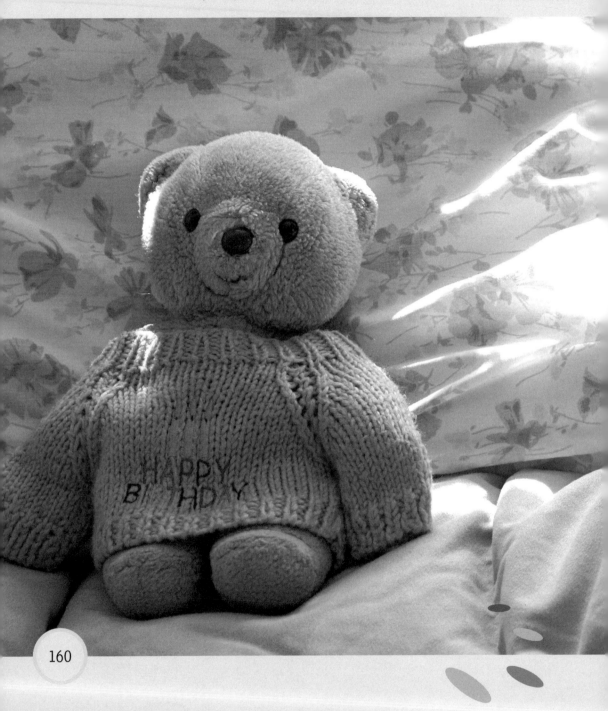

37

Mattress matters

Is your bed soft or lumpy? Have you had it for over 15 years? It may be time to look for a new one.

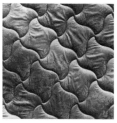

Just how comfortable is your bed? Do you disappear under the mattress or maybe you and your bed partner end up in a dip in the middle of the bed? One study found that replacing an uncomfortable bed led to an increase of 42 minutes' sleep.

Did you know that beds should be replaced every eight to ten years, by which time they've deteriorated by as much as 75% – yet the average couple hang on to their haven of slumber for fifteen years or more? This can not only lead to back pain, it can mean you're tossing and turning all night trying to get into a comfortable position. The result? You wake up in the night, you don't sleep so soundly, your sleep time is cut short and you feel groggy the next day.

To relieve and prevent back pain you need a bed with the correct support and comfort. The idea is to keep your spine in correct alignment, while the bed moulds itself to your natural body contours. This will also mean you'll be moving around less,

Here's an idea for you...

Go into a shop with a list of your priorities and concerns in advance – health, size, storage, price and so on. There are so many different types of bed that you could be tempted by something you don't really need. Narrow your choice down to two or three and then spend plenty of time – with your partner if you have one – lying on these in your normal sleeping positions. Five or ten minutes should be the minimum for each bed – but feel free to spend half an hour, though any longer and you'll be in danger of settling down for the night.

too. Remember, you're going to spend over 29,000 hours on your bed during an average lifespan so it's worth taking a little time and effort to make the right choice.

BEFORE YOU BUY ...

■ Consider a bigger bed. People just don't buy large enough beds. Three-quarters of all double beds are still the standard 4ft 6in × 6ft 3in (135 × 190cm) – yet this is plainly not room enough for two adults to sleep comfortably together without disturbing each other. Studies have shown that couples sleep better in a bigger bed – on average we prod each other 120 times a night. No wonder the Victorians favoured separate bedrooms. If that's not an option, go for size. The standard 4ft 6in × 6ft 3in (135 × 190cm) is still the most popular size, but over a quarter of us opt for bigger beds. Even upgrading to the next size, a 5ft/150cm king size, whilst it takes up very little extra bedroom space, makes a considerable difference! Most shops now have 6ft (180cm) beds too.

■ Look for a supportive rather than a hard bed – gone are the days when people thought you needed a hard bed for a good night's sleep. The modern view is that correct support (which is dependent on your weight and build) coupled with comfort is best. Don't automatically go for an orthopaedic bed either – often a medium firm bed with proper cushioning is better.

- Look at pocket spring beds – they tend to feel softer, as they are packed with more upholstery and also feature smaller, lighter springs than a conventional mattress. Because they have so many springs packed tightly together, they give good individual support.

- Consider a waterbed. Forget 70s sex comedies, waterbeds can seriously improve your sleep. Just lying on a waterbed is a relaxing experience – it's like floating and you get a feeling of weightlessness. Most waterbeds have a heater, so you can choose a temperature to suit you. They also conform perfectly to your body, so you're less likely to move around.

- Get a space bed – well, a foam mattresses based on NASA technology. The mattress stops tossing and turning by moulding to the shape and position of your body. On an uncomfortable bed, your body needs to change position because of unrelieved pressure. Your blood flow is restricted and there's a build up of pressure – this makes you uncomfortable and forces your body to reposition. When your spine is supported in the correct anatomical shape, there's less pressure build up and therefore less tossing and turning.

You're happy with your bed – now make sure your bedroom is up to scratch. Turn it into a quiet, relaxing sanctuary by taking a look at IDEA 38, *Snoozy rooms*.

Try another idea...

'My dream would be to work from my bed – a big bed with eternally fresh sheets – so that I could doze off whenever I wanted to and work in between.'

ANNA RAEBURN

Defining idea...

Q   When should I buy a new bed?

A   *Don't wait until your bed is uncomfortable or damaged before replacing it, by which time your sleep quality could be quite severely affected – use other triggers. Even a good-quality bed will only last around 10 years.*

Q   I want to buy a pocket spring mattress but the ones I have seen seem lumpy. Will it be comfortable?

A   *Yes. Luxury, pocket spring beds don't have flat surfaces – they mould themselves to your body shape and the indentation remains even if you turn the bed regularly.*

Q   What kind of pillow should I look for?

A   *Choose a pillow which supports your neck and make sure it lines up with the rest of the spine. Too many pillows thrust the head forward or sideways (depending on your sleeping position) which can create a crick in the neck.*

38

Snoozy rooms

If your bedroom is giving off the wrong signals, you could find yourself livening up again – then your mind will start racing and you'll find it impossible to drop off.

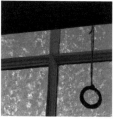

The key is to turn your bedroom into a quiet, relaxing place that you associate with sleep and sex rather than somewhere that resembles an office or, even worse, a nightclub.

CREATE A LUXURIOUS OASIS

If you dread going to bed because you have too much to do or have difficulty falling asleep, try making bedtime seem more luxurious so you'll look forward to it. For example, invest in cotton sheets with a high thread count (at least 200 threads per inch); they cost more but feel softer. Change your bedding about once a week, or often enough to keep it feeling fresh.

Scenting your bedroom with fragrant herbs can also make bedtime feel special – but remember less is more. You don't want your bedroom smelling like a cheap perfume counter. Try stuffing a couple of tablespoons of dried lavender in a small cloth bag and tucking it among your pillows. This acts as a mild sedative, too.

Here's an idea for you... **Take an inventory of everything in your bedroom from the pictures you've got on the wall to the piles of magazines in the corner – then give it marks out of ten according to how stimulating it is and whether you think it stops you from going to sleep. You should remove from your bedroom everything that scores over 5 out of 10. Your sound system and CD collection, for instance, may get 8. Listening to loud, pounding music before bed is not a good idea – your body will gear itself up for a night of dancing, not dozing.**

Remove distractions. Your bedroom environment should calm you. That means no computers, CD players and television or piles of books, magazines, letters, bills and dirty clothes, which can all make you feel anxious and keep you awake. If you must keep electronics in your bedroom, at least turn them off before bedtime and keep them out of your line of sight. You could even cover them with a cloth. And you might have to get rid of that huge photo of New York hanging in your bedroom. Visual distractions like pictures remain in your mind even after you've turned out the lights.

Block out light. For the best quality sleep, make your room as dark as possible. Too much light and your body won't make enough of the hormone melatonin. This helps regulate your sleep cycle, sending you off to sleep and helping you stay that way. The amount of light you're exposed to at any given moment is what tells the pineal gland in your brain whether or not to produce melatonin. The darker it is when you sleep, the better your melatonin production, and the better the quality of your sleep. To block out light from outside always draw your blinds or curtains

– and ideally invest in blackout versions which let in virtually no light. And turn brightly lit digital clocks around so you can't see them.

Choose the right temperature. Most sleep scientists believe that a slightly cool room contributes to good sleep – about 60 to 65 degrees Fahrenheit (16 to 18 degrees Celsius). That's because it matches what occurs deep inside the body, when the body's internal temperature drops during the night to its lowest level. (For good sleepers, this occurs about four hours after they begin sleeping.) Everyone's body temperature is set slightly differently because it changes according to your body clock. And if you've got insomnia your body temperature won't fluctuate as much as in normal sleepers. Body temperature patterns also change with age, and are related to changes in sleep patterns. As you get older, your body temperatures start to rise and fall earlier – which leads to less sleep. Two people with different body temperatures are obviously going to disagree about the desired sleep temperature. It's still best to turn the thermostat down at night in cold weather – it not only saves on your fuel bills, it sets the stage for your sleep. If your bed partner is feeling cold, replace your duvet with blankets that can be piled on and taken off as you wish. Your other half may benefit from an electric blanket or warmer bedclothes. Bed socks aren't the most glamorous of night attire, but they definitely work.

To find out how your bedroom can make you richer and improve your relationship as well as give you a good night's sleep, check out IDEA 40, *The* feng shui *bedroom*.

Try another idea…

'For sleep, one needs endless depths of blackness to sink into; daylight is too shallow, it will not cover one.'
ANNE MORROW LINDBERGH,
author and wife of aviator
Charles Lindbergh

Defining idea…

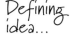

Q   Just how dark should it be?

A   *As dark as possible. Even dim light from a night-light or hall light can dis-*
rupt sleep cycles and prevent you from getting deep sleep. Research has
shown that if you can see your hand after all the lights are out, then it's
light enough to affect the gland that produces melatonin.

Q   I often wake up with a sore throat. Could my bedroom be to
blame?

A   *The air in your bedroom could be too dry. Other signs of too little humidity*
include dryness in your nose or even a nose bleed. So consider a humidi-
fier or leave out a bowl of boiling water when you get into bed. If you also
suffer with an itchy throat or watery eyes, you could be allergic to some-
thing in the bedroom such as dust mites, the microscopic creatures that live
by the millions in mattresses and bedding. Wash your bedding weekly in
hot water and use mite-proof mattress and pillow covers to prevent expo-
sure to mite waste and fragments.

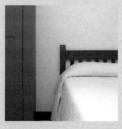

39

What a racket!

Whether you're being kept awake by noisy neighbours or people playing loud music in their cars outside, think about noiseproofing your bedroom.

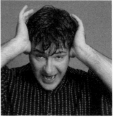

You're lying in bed, and you're ready to drop off, when suddenly you hear the neighbours start an argument about where they're going on holiday. Not again. It's the third time this week and it's seriously disrupting your sleep.

First, some basic advice. Timber floorboards make noise reverberate around the room – so consider fitting carpets or thick rugs to stop this. Close windows and doors when you want peace and quiet and fill in any gaps in seals which will let in noise. And fit heavy curtains across large windows which help keep noise out. If you're still being disturbed by the noise, you'll have to try something more extreme.

Test how well soundproofed your windows are. Seal gaps with plasticine, which can be removed without damaging paint surfaces. This should be tested for several days and nights. If noise levels go down, think about fitting sealing devices on your windows which allow your windows to be open, while maximising noise reduction when they're closed. The seals need to be fitted by a skilled DIY person – it has to be done carefully to block all gaps, while still allowing the window to open with enough resistance.

WINDOWS AND WALLS

Windows are the most common way for noise to get in. Single glass panes and wood window frames are the least resistant to noise. Fitting your window frames with thicker glass can help – twice as thick and your traffic noise will drop by half. Double glazing can reduce noise by about 20%, while vinyl frames can reduce it by 50%.

If you don't want to pay for new glass or frames, consider a removable plug to block the sound coming through the window. This is a soundproofing board made from special soundproofing material which you place over your window before you go to bed. It also blocks light, but who cares if it stops all the noise that's keeping you awake? It's dark anyway. And the extra insulation of a plug will keep you warmer in winter and cooler in summer. Unless you've got a first-class honours degree in DIY I recommend you get an expert to do this one. A plug is made by measuring the window frame and seeing how much depth there is to the window sill. This will determine the size and thickness of the soundproofing material you can use – whoever is making it for you will go to a DIY store for soundproofing materials. The soundproofing mat is usually about two inches (5cm) thick. While the mat is relatively stiff, it can be attached to a lightweight wood or plasterboard using contact cement. A plug should fit a window very tightly without any cracks. For easy handling, your builder may attach some handles to it.

As well as reducing your central heating bill, insulating your bedroom wall will reduce the amount of noise that's let in. If you're trying to block out the noise coming from your street, you only really need to soundproof that wall. The best way to do this is by dry lining, where the wall is lined with insulating material and covered in plasterboard.

Your bedroom may be quiet now, but if it's filled with clutter you're still going to have trouble switching off. For tips on clearing the clutter and creating a peaceful, relaxing environment, take a look at IDEA 38, *Snoozy rooms*. To find out how to arrange your bedroom to boost your health and well-being, check out IDEA 40, *The* feng shui bedroom.

Try another idea…

THE ATTIC

Many attics, especially in older homes, have no insulation. Putting it in not only cuts down on your heating bills, it can also help to soundproof your home. Extra layers of tarmac can also increase your home's noise tolerance, especially to aircraft. If you live near an airport, try stapling extra tarmac sheets on the roof rafters inside the attic – it's a cheap and effective way to reduce noise.

'He who sleeps in continual noise is wakened by silence.'
WILLIAM DEAN HOWELLS,
American novelist

Defining idea…

Q **Does the type of door you have make any difference to the amount of sound let in?**

A *A hollow door will always let in more sound than a solid one. And make sure you fill in any gaps in the seals.*

Q **I can hear people walking around upstairs when I go to sleep. They're not doing anything antisocial like playing loud music, but it still keeps me awake. What can I do to block the sound?**

A *The people living above you probably have floorboards. Maybe you could write a polite note to your landlord if you're all renting, telling them about the noise. Or chat to them about it yourself. Simply putting down a large rug could reduce the noise dramatically. Experts say that at least 25% of a room should have some absorbent material, like carpeting or furniture, to reduce reverberation from footsteps. If your neighbours refuse to cooperate or you can still hear the noise, think about getting a builder to install a suspended plasterboard ceiling. This should block out most noise from above.*

Q **Is there anything you can do outside the house to stop the noise coming in?**

A *Some soundproofing experts suggest putting up a barrier between the noise source and your bedroom window. This could be a fence, screen or garden feature that will block the path of the soundwaves.*

40

The *feng shui* bedroom

Pick up some slumber tips from this ancient Chinese philosophy.

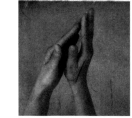

Feng shui makes some pretty incredible claims about bedrooms: the way you arrange it can affect not only your sleep but your relationships, your bank balance and your health.

Whatever your views, anything that promises to make you richer, livelier, brimming with vitality and happier in your marriage as well give you a good night's sleep is worth investigating …

The idea behind *feng shui* – pronounced fung shway – is to increase harmony in your environment. *Chi* is the invisible life force that is in everything around us. Sometimes, *chi* moves too quickly, too slowly, or is stopped in its tracks. This results in bad energy, which can ruin your sleep, relationships and health. Anyway, have fun checking out these tips on keeping a good flow of *chi*. Don't feel you have to do them all – just try to create a warm, cosy, uncluttered space.

Here's an idea for you... **If you really want to use white paint in your bedroom but are worried about draining the room's energy, you can always add splashes of bright red. Chinese believe that red brings luck and red is used for healing, wealth, strength and vitality. Red curtains, a red throw or red cushions on your bed will boost the energy in your room.**

GET THE BASICS

If you have a choice of rooms, go for one that's towards the back of your house where it's quieter. *Feng shui* regards bedrooms as private sanctuaries for romance and restoration. Be clear what your bedroom is for and take out anything that doesn't fit this goal – that means computers, televisions, a desk and even your dirty laundry basket. Stale energy hangs around dirty laundry. Remove any other clutter – under your bed, for instance – as this is meant to indicate there's clutter in your relationship. Any furniture should be comfortable and safe with rounded or soft edges and corners.

Place your bed correctly, with the head against a solid wall so that when you're in it you feel safe and secure. And never put your bed under a window– according to *feng shui* principles, this may lead to a lack of support from those around you. The rush of *chi* from the window could also cause restless sleep. You shouldn't place your bed under an exposed beam either. Apparently, sleeping under a beam causes ill health, bad luck and relationship problems such as back-stabbing and jealousy. Lastly, do not place your bed with the head or foot pointed at a door. This is known as the coffin position, and it drains away all your good luck and energy. Ideally, the bed should be within sight of the door but off to one side. This promotes restful sleep and, according to *feng shui*, keeps negative forces from entering the room while you sleep.

THINK ABOUT ACCESSORIES

Pairs of candlesticks, vases or picture frames are thought to increase marital harmony. Putting nightstands and lights on both sides of the bed invites your partner into your nest. If you want to hang pictures, opt for landscape posters of warm sunsets or grassy fields.

Go for the shine – mirrors and anything that reflects or shines light such as crystals, chandeliers, lamps, reflective surfaces and shiny ribbons are key ingredients in a *feng shui* bedroom. They are meant to bounce energy in different directions. A chandelier is useful because crystals absorb bad energy, and also add light. So add a mirror, a big chandelier, a couple of sparkly lamps and a few shiny bowls and hopefully you and your partner will be enjoying harmonious evenings in your bedroom, chatting and laughing, followed by energetic sex and the best night's sleep you've ever had.

Give your bedroom a coat of paint, because adding colour to a room is a great way to get rid of bad energy. White is associated with death and mourning and drains energy, so pick colours like cream or antique white if you want a neutral colour. Or try pale pastels like peach, lemon or pink.

Is your bed lumpy, bumpy, squashy or spongy? Find out if it's time to get a new bed in IDEA 37, *Mattress matters*. For more conventional tips on making your bedroom an enjoyable place to sleep, check out IDEA 38, *Snoozy rooms*.

Try another idea...

'Many successful people already practice some form of feng shui without actually realising it.'

THE FENG SHUI SOCIETY

Defining idea...

Q What about bed sheets – should they be pastel shades too?

A *Yes, they should – unless you've been feeling lethargic lately, in which case red bed sheets could pep you up. Pink bedding is thought to help relationships, green encourages family harmony, healing, vitality and a new start, yellow is for health, purple for wealth and blue for knowledge.*

Q You say get rid of computers, but I've heard that they create energy. Is this true?

A *It's true that some modern feng shui practitioners use electric items such as computers, radio and TV sets to help the flow of chi. If a room is lifeless and empty, they say, turning on the radio or the computer can create energy. But this doesn't work for everyone.*

Q My friend, who follows *feng shui*, has chimes in her room. I'm sure the sound of clanking chimes would irritate me – if not my husband. Do they really work?

A *Wind chimes create harmonious sounds and movement and increase the flow of good energy as a result. If you're not enthusiastic about the prospect of chimes hanging over your bed, and think it would be a source of tension rather than harmony in your relationship, you could opt for a less intrusive option – a mobile. They create the same effect, but without the danger of being woken up by irritating tinklings.*

41

Music to my ears

From whale music to Mozart, how to turn on, tune in, drop off ...

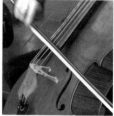

Music is powerful and can actually have physiological effects — from improving your mood to lowering your heart rate. And one study found that 96% of people's sleep improved after listening to classical or new age music. So now's your chance to build your very own compilation of snoozy tracks.

You put on your favourite track – what's happening to your body? The sound goes in through your ear which sends impulses to the brain. Your brain reacts to these impulses and sends out directions that help control your heart rate, breathing, blood pressure and muscle tension. Music can even trigger the painkilling, mood-boosting chemicals endorphins. The right track can therefore slow your breathing and your heart rate, relax your muscles and put you in a great mood. If that's not a recipe for a good night's sleep, I don't know what is.

Here's an idea for you... **Find out how music affects your heart rate. Test it by listening to various pieces of music, fast and slow, and then taking your own pulse. Your heart will speed up or slow down to match the rhythm of a sound so if you're listening to a slower piece, your heart will beat slower to match it.**

So what music should you be listening to and will this mean that you have to destroy your collection of heavy metal? Probably. Most say that music to relax you before bed should be quiet, melodic with a slow beat and few, if any, rhythmic accents. Listening to Pachelbel's Canon, for instance, at around 64 beats per minute, the rate of a resting heart beat, will slow your breathing rate and heart rate and change your brainwave pattern from rapid beta waves to the slower, sleepier alpha ones. And Mozart, which contains a lot of high notes, seems to reduce the level of adrenaline and slow the metabolism.

HOW TO USE MUSIC EFFECTIVELY

- Turn your mood around – make a happy tape. Find three songs that sound like you feel when you're stressed or down, three that feel like you want to feel and three in between. Then record them on to a tape. The music should gradually become calmer, quieter and slower. Put this on in the evening and it will guide you through your feelings and lift your mood.

- Let someone else do the work for you. There are hundreds of relaxation CDs on the market – some simply for relaxing, some for insomnia and stress. If you don't fancy music, look to nature – you can now get anything from whale and dolphin music to the sounds of waterfalls and waves crashing against the shore. If you're feeling adventurous, make your own tape of relaxing sounds – walking through autumn leaves, running water, tweeting birds ...

- Try sound therapy. This is the theory that toning – making a sound with an elongated vowel for an extended period – can help relieve tension and relax your muscles. Apparently, every organ in our body has a certain vibration, which can get out of balance – and hitting the right note can restore the balance. For a three-minute relaxation, make a long-o (as in ocean) or ah (as in aha) sound. This helps get rid of any thoughts cluttering your mind. If the sounds of waterfalls and twittering birds aren't up your street, then you're better off playing something you like. Not everyone responds to classical music, but anything that you enjoy and find relaxing that pushes other noises, like traffic, out of your mind is going to help you sleep. If that's thrash metal or heavy rock, then so be it. If you play a piece of music that you don't like – even if it is classical – then it won't be restful. And if a slow tune gives your mind time to fret or obsess, it's a waste of time – you need something livelier to distract you.
- Once you've chosen your music, lie down quietly, taking even, deep breaths. Try to clear your head of all your thoughts. Just let the music wash over you. Keep listening when you get to bed. Your heart rate should lower, metabolism drop, eyelids droopy, sleep.

Put on your favourite uplifting music while you perform the invigorating stretching routine in IDEA 49, Wake-up stretches.

Try another idea...

'Why waste money on psychotherapy when you can listen to the B Minor Mass?'

MICHAEL TORKE, composer

Defining idea...

Q **I've heard about music that copies your brainwaves to help you get to sleep. Do you know where I could get hold of it?**

A Yes, Canadian researchers have made individually tailored brain music to help insomnia – but it's not yet available. They've created music which matches a person's brainwaves and when played lowers their anxiety levels so they're able to relax and sleep. The computer programme that comes up with the healing music creates the same brain patterns you have when you're meditating. So when you go to sleep the same brainwave patterns are triggered. You can already buy CDs out there that generally replicate the brainwaves – but tailor-made tapes are obviously going to be more effective.

Q **I had no idea that vibrations from sound waves can also have a direct impact on individual body parts. Is there scientific backing?**

A Yes, to a certain extent. Scientists have long known that every atom vibrates, emitting sound waves even though they're far too faint for us to hear. Since body parts are made up of atoms, they all produce sound waves. Some therapists believe that these sound waves are altered when disease or stress hits – and they also believe that directing sound waves at the body or its parts (by chanting certain sounds) can restore natural rhythms and encourage healing.

42

Say yes to yoga

Need to learn how to relax before bedtime? Perform a 20-minute yoga routine and you'll not only feel less stressed, but your body will feel relaxed and floppy too.

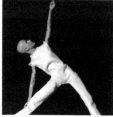

And some experts claim half an hour of yoga can actually reduce the amount of sleep you need each night. What are you waiting for? Grab your yoga mat and begin ...

Yoga uses a series of poses, breathing and meditative techniques that relax you and calm your nervous system. That's why it's perfect for people with sleep problems. Once you're regularly practising yoga, you'll fall asleep in a shorter time – mainly because your body and mind are more relaxed. The quality of your sleep will improve because of yoga's beneficial effect on the nervous system, and in particular the brain. As a result, you may even need less sleep.

FIRST 10 MINUTES – JUST BREATHE

The key to all yoga is breathing. By learning how to slow your rate of breathing, you shed yourself of the day's stresses that have made your muscles tense and have filled your mind with worries. This may take weeks of practice so you'll have to do

Here's an idea for you...

Taking you a while to master slow breathing? Try a simpler alternative called 2–1 breathing. You can even do this one in bed. Gently slow down the rate of exhalation until you exhale for twice as long as you inhale. Don't try to fill or empty the lungs completely – you are simply changing the rhythm of your breath. It may help to count to six on the exhalation and three on the inhalation, or four on the exhalation and two on the inhalation (or any other 2 to 1 ratio you find comfortable). Your breath should flow smoothly, evenly and continuously. When you've mastered it take 8 breaths lying on your back, 16 breaths on your right side and 32 on your left side.

it in the day until you can use it before you go to bed. Sit or stand where you can see a clock. Put your hands on your lower ribs and count the number of times you breathe in and out normally in one minute. The average is 14–16 times. Then breathe slightly faster than usual and count the breaths (in and out) that you take in one minute. Finally, take a break to calm your breathing, then repeat the exercise, this time trying to breathe much more slowly than you normally do. With practice, you should be able to slow your rate of breathing to as few as six breaths a minute – the usual rate during meditation.

NEXT 10 MINUTES – THE POSES

Now try some calming poses such as forward bends and twists. Simple inversions such as lying with your feet up the wall also help you unwind. The child's pose, however, will probably make you want to drop off immediately. Kneel down and sit on your feet with your heels pointing outward. Your knees should be separated, about the width of your hips. Place your forehead on the floor, then bring your arms alongside your body, palms turned upward. Stay for about three minutes. To come up from the child's pose, lengthen the front of your body then inhale as you lift from your tailbone, pressing down and into your pelvis.

LAST 5 MINUTES – RELAX

Finally, do the corpse pose. Lie on your back, with your feet spread about 18 inches (45cm) apart, your hands about 6 inches (15cm) from your sides, palms up. Let your thighs, knees and toes turn outward. Close your eyes and breathe deeply. Then first tense then relax each part of your body in turn, working up from your feet to your head.

Do you find it easier doing your yoga when you're listening to music? Look at IDEA 41, *Music to my ears*, to find out the best sounds to put on.

Try another idea…

If you wake up in the middle of the night and find it difficult to drop back off then you could try the bridge pose. You'll have to get out of bed for this, but it works. You lie on your back, bend your knees and set your feet on the floor, heels as close to your bottom as possible. Breathe out and, pressing your feet and arms into the floor, push up your pelvis, lifting your bottom off the floor. Clasp your hands below your pelvis and extend through the arms to help you stay on the tops of your shoulders. Lift your bottom until your thighs are about parallel to the floor. Firm your outer arms, broaden your shoulder blades, and try to lift the space between them at the base of the neck up into your body. Stay in the pose anywhere from 30 seconds to 1 minute. Release with an exhalation, rolling your spine slowly down onto the floor.

'Tension is who you think you should be. Relaxation is who you are.'

CHINESE PROVERB

Defining idea…

183

How did it go?

Q Should I do back bends as well as forward bends?

A *In general, back bends are stimulating, while forward bends are calming. If you overemphasise back bends or perform them with misalignment, then you could stimulate your adrenals and will be full of energy rather than relaxed when you try to go to sleep.*

Q Is any particular type of yoga better for sleep?

A *Most of the moves I have mentioned come from hatha yoga – the type of yoga most widely used in the West. Hatha means balance and combines postures with breathing. However, there are many kinds of yoga – some, like astanga, are more energising so wouldn't be so good at bedtime and others like raja focus on meditation. Before you go to sleep, you obviously need to stick to calming poses. You may need to talk to a yoga specialist to get a programme designed for you.*

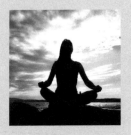

43

Ommmm ...

Use meditation to rid yourself of information overload and clear your head for bed.

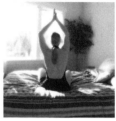

Forget kaftans, long beards and headscarves, meditation has moved into the twenty-first century. From Hollywood stars to executives and busy mums, people everywhere are using meditation to solve their sleep problems. So chill out, unwind and relax.

If you can't switch off in the evening and your babbling thoughts are keeping you awake at night, learning to meditate may well be the answer. Fans say that meditating helps you to rise above everyday niggles and sort out what's important to you. It can even help you solve problems. Scientists have backed this up – do it regularly, and the levels of your stress hormones will plummet as will your blood levels of lactic acid, which is associated with anxiety. Blood pressure – another symptom of a stressful lifestyle – also goes down.

Got no time? Try this two-minute relaxation meditation. Sit comfortably with your spine reasonably straight. Allow your eyes to rest comfortably downward, not focused on anything. Without closing your eyes completely, let your eyelids drop to a level that feels relaxed and comfortable. Continue gazing down – the act of gazing is your primary focus rather than the area at which you are gazing. You may notice your breathing gradually becoming more rhythmic. It's OK to let your attention drift a bit. If your eyes become very heavy then let them close.

You don't really need much to meditate – just a blanket and a mat for comfort and loose-fitting clothing. And you might like to listen to music to help you unwind initially. Sit comfortably with your back straight, either in a chair or on the floor, with your eyes closed. If you're worried about whether you're sitting correctly, just make sure you're comfortable and that you're back is straight. If you want to sit like the pros, however, try the seven point posture. Sit with your legs crossed. If you're supple try the half or full-lotus posture in which one or both feet are placed soles upward on the thigh of the opposite leg. Then place both hands in your lap, right hand above the left, palms upward and with thumbs touching. Your back should be kept straight but with your head tilted forward slightly. Your eyes may either be completely closed or left a fraction open. Your mouth should be loosely closed.

Now breathe deeply. Bring your breath right down to your navel and, as you exhale, let go of any bad feelings and feel the day's stresses and worries drift away. Tell yourself that with each breath you're becoming more and more relaxed. Your brainwaves will now have slowed down to levels associated with stage 1 sleep. The more you practice, the better you'll get at reaching a state of total calm. Aim for two 20-minute sessions a day – ideally once before breakfast and once in the evening.

WHICH ONE'S FOR YOU?

There are different types of meditation, but all follow the same principle – focusing your mind on one image, word or abstract idea. Here are the main three …

If you find it difficult to get started, you might find it easier to put on some music. Check out IDEA 41, *Music to my ears*, for some tune choices.

Try another idea…

- Transcendental meditation (TM). When practicing TM, you repeat a mantra to yourself throughout the meditation. A teacher may give you the mantra or you may simply use a word that is calming to you, such as peace or sea. Saying the mantra helps prevent distracting thoughts from entering your mind and allows you to gradually relax and release stress. The idea is to reach a passive state where thoughts, images and feelings pass through your consciousness almost unnoticed.
- Mindfulness meditation. Allow all your thoughts and feelings to come and go but don't react to them – this is a way of letting go of worries about work, children and relationships. In a similar way you can do a body scan, where you think about each part of your body from head to toe. As you let go of thoughts or images associated with each body part, the body part lets go, too, thus releasing much of its tension. As well as relaxation, it's great for cramps, restless legs syndrome and any other pain that could be keeping you awake. For best results, a body scan should take about 45 minutes.
- Breath meditation. This involves focusing on breathing in and breathing out – you should try not to let your thoughts shift from your breath. Concentrating on something as basic as the breath helps to clear your mind.

'Meditation is like bubble bath for the soul – you can sink into it at any time and it'll make you feel great.'

THE BAREFOOT DOCTOR

Defining idea…

187

How did it go?

Q   Can you learn how to meditate at home?

A   *Yes it's possible. You may need to go on a course to learn transcendental meditation, but other forms of yoga, which include meditation techniques, can be picked up from books, videos or DVDs. Compare prices too – many TM schools charge a lot for the practices they teach.*

Q   Do you have to be religious to meditate?

A   *No, it's a technique. That said, meditation is associated with some religions such as Buddhism and Hinduism. And some transcendental meditation courses have more religious overtones than others, so shop around to make sure you're comfortable with the philosophy.*

Q   I don't have time to meditate. What should I do?

A   *The busier you are, the more you need meditation. You'll be surprised how much time you're wasting already worrying about things you don't need to or fretting over something but not doing anything about it. Meditation, however, will help you sort out your priorities so you'll end up having more time. And you'll sleep better, so you'll be more alert too. Set aside a time for meditation to make it a habit. Aim for 20 minutes in the morning and evening, but if you can do only one, then so be it.*

44

Herb power

If you thought herbs were simply for adding flavour to soups and casseroles, think again.

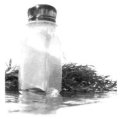

They're pretty powerful stuff and in the right quantities, herbs can help you beat insomnia — particularly if it's caused by stress and anxiety. So put on the kettle, make a lavender tea and read on ...

Like conventional drugs, herbs cause straightforward biochemical reactions in your body. In fact, many of today's drugs are based on substances found in herbs. But unlike most conventional drugs, herbalism uses all of the plant (the root, stem or leaf) in a variety of ways – from pills and teas to tinctures, which are concentrates made by leaving the herb in alcohol.

So how can herbs improve your sleep? Sleep disorders and depression are linked with an imbalance in the brain chemical serotonin, which your body makes from the amino acid tryptophan. Certain herbs can help restore proper serotonin levels in the brain. Other herbs work by triggering your brain's calming chemicals.

Grow your own lavender. This is one of the easiest herbs to grow. Buy seeds from your local garden centre – look for the name Lavandula angustifolia – and plant them indoors on trays until they're ready to be replanted in a pot, windowbox or the garden. Feed regularly with organic plant food. During the growing season, late spring to mid autumn, regularly soak the soil and keep a daily lookout for pests – spray insects with a solution of liquid soap. As soon as they flower, cut the leaves from the stems, tie in loose bunches and leave suspended in a warm dry place until completely dry. Store in an airtight jar. Then prune your lavender plant – ready for next year.

You can buy herbs from health food shops and chemists or, if you've got green fingers, you can even grow your own – all you need is a windowbox. Just stick to the recommended doses as some herbs can be pretty potent. Alternatively, consult a practitioner – preferably someone who's been recommended to you or is a member of a respected professional association.

The quality of herbs varies among manufacturers. Poor-quality herbs may contain contaminants or only small amounts of active ingredients, so always ask your practitioner for assurances on safety and quality. They should be able to tell you the name of the supplier and all products should be clearly labelled and ideally have a batch number. This usually means that the batch has been checked for quality and ensures that it can be traced back to source if there are any problems.

HERBS THAT HELP YOU SLEEP

- *Chamomile*. Your grandmother was probably a big believer in chamomile tea. And she was right. Studies have found chamomile has a sedative effect – and unlike some herbs it's safe for pregnant and breastfeeding women. Put it in your bath in the evening. To make a calming tea, add one teaspoon of the flower to boiling water and steep in the pan – with the lid on – for five to ten minutes.

If you like herbs, you'll love aromatherapy oils. Turn to IDEA 46, *It makes scents*, for the best oils to use and how to use them.

Try another idea...

- *Hops.* Yes, it's the same hops that's in beer but no, it doesn't mean you can have a pint before bedtime. Instead, fill a pillow with dried hops – a traditional remedy for sleeplessness and nervous conditions. Tea made from hops is an acquired taste – it's pretty bitter, but a spoonful of honey can take the edge off it. You can also buy freeze-dried extract in capsule form.

- *Lavender.* One of the most calming herbs, lavender will help you deal with stress-related insomnia. Make a calming tincture of the herb by steeping it in vodka for a month, then straining. Take a teaspoonful three times a day until your tension lifts. Or make a sachet of lavender to leave under your pillow at night. For headaches, rub the essential oil on your temples.

- *Lemon balm.* Also known as melissa, lemon balm is a sedative and stomach-soother often used in combination with other sedative herbs. Add 2 or 3 teaspoons of the dried herb to a cup of freshly boiled water and let it steep for 5 to 15 minutes for a soothing tea that actually tastes nice too.

- *Valerian.* This speeds up the time it takes to get to sleep and reduces night-time waking – without the hangover-type side effects of Valium and other synthetic sedatives. Put 2 to 3 droppersful of tincture made from fresh valerian roots (or 1 to 2 teaspoons of dried valerian root) in hot water for a bedtime drink. Take no more than one cup a day – too much can cause headaches.

- *St John's wort* (Hypericum perforatum). Studies show that it can help relieve

'And still she slept an azure-lidded sleep,
In blanched linen, smooth, and lavender'd.'

JOHN KEATS

Defining idea...

chronic insomnia and mild depression when they're due to an imbalance in brain chemistry. It's most commonly taken in capsule form.

How did it go?

Q Are there any side effects with herbal medicine?

A *Although herbs are considered natural alternatives to certain drugs and for the most part have a good safety record, they can be equally powerful, as well as toxic. That's why it's vital to read the label when you're buying herbs or consult a knowledgeable herbal expert. You should also consult your doctor before taking any herbal remedy – particularly if you're pregnant or breastfeeding. Some have side effects when combined with medicines. St John's wort, for instance, can make the contraceptive pill less effective. And kava kava reacts badly with some antidepressants.*

Q What should I expect when I see a herbalist?

A *During your first consultation you'll be quizzed about your lifestyle and health background such as your diet, work and emotional life. You may have a physical examination much like a doctor would do for a basic medical and you'll need to give details of any medical prescriptions you're taking. Remedies are made up on the spot, and you may be asked to come back in a week or two.*

45

The sweetest pill

Forget the 'placebo effect', homeopathy is now a respected way to treat sleep problems.

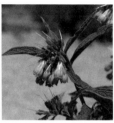

It doesn't just treat insomnia, though, it treats your particular type of insomnia and takes into account the time you wake up, your personality and even what you had for lunch last Thursday.

Homeopaths believe that symptoms are a sign of your body trying to heal itself. The remedies aim to stimulate your immune system and other healing mechanisms. As you probably already know, the idea is to treat like with like: you use a remedy that would produce similar symptoms to the ones you're suffering from if it were taken in full strength. For example, under normal circumstances a cup of coffee would make you alert and give your mind a buzz. So you take the homeopathic remedy, coffea, when your mind is overactive to help you switch off before bedtime.

The remedies are tiny amounts of substances from plants, minerals and animal products and are prepared by a long process of shaking and dilution until finally not a single molecule of the original substance remains. In fact, the more diluted

Here's an idea for you… **If you buy over-the-counter remedies, log the effects of each remedy you try in a homeopathy diary. Take only one remedy at a time and move on to the next remedy after a few weeks if you're not happy with the results. Remember not to touch the remedies when you take them as this can interfere with the results – empty them onto a teaspoon and put it under your tongue or put them in the cap of the bottle, then tip them into your mouth. And store your remedies in a cool dark place in a tightly closed bottle away from strong smells such as perfumes or essential oils. Stored correctly, remedies will keep for around five years.**

a remedy, the more potent it is – so a 30c remedy is stronger than a 6c remedy. Most remedies come in tablet form.

You can buy remedies from chemists and health shops but ideally you should consult a homeopath first to ensure you're taking the right one for your symptoms and your personality type. The remedies are unbelievably specific and can take into account everything from how tall you are, whether you're an irritable person or an organiser to whether you've got a good memory or have a sense of humour. The personality bit may seem a bit odd, but homeopaths believe that symptoms do not occur in isolation, but are an overall reflection of a person. They therefore don't just look at the problem presented to them but at the person as a whole. That means considering a patient's personality, temperament, emotional and physical state and likes and dislikes before prescribing a treatment. So a homeopath might see two people with similar symptoms, but would treat them totally differently.

You normally take a remedy an hour before going to bed and for up to 14 days. And if you wake up in the night and can't get back to sleep, you can repeat the dose.

DOZY DOSES

- Nux vomica – for when you wake up around 3 or 4 in the morning because you've eaten too much the night before or had too much alcohol. You fall asleep just as it's time to get up and are in a bad mood all day. It suits mainly men, competitive types, people who are critical but can't take criticism from others and those who like rich fatty food.

- Pulsatilla – for when you're restless in the early hours of sleep and you just can't get comfortable. It suits mainly women, good natured and emotional types, those who prefer sweet food.

- Arnica – for when your bed feels too hard and you are overtired and fidgety. It suits imaginative people and those who put off going to the doctor.

- Lycopodium – for when your mind is active before bed and you're unable to get rid of thoughts about work. You dream a lot and wake up around 4 in the morning. It suits people who are tall and lean, dislike change and are prone to exaggeration.

- Arsenicum – for when you wake up between midnight and 2 in the morning feeling restless and worried. It suits a person who has strong ideas, is attentive to detail and likes everything in its place.

- Rhus tox – for when you can't sleep and feel a need to walk about or you suffer from restless legs syndrome. It suits those who are lively and anxious at night.

Try another idea...

Other therapies that look at the whole person when treating sleep problems include acupuncture and aromatherapy – to find out more, take a look at IDEA 47, *Get to the point* and IDEA 46, *It makes scents.*

Defining idea...

'You take the blue pill, the story ends. You wake up in your bed and you believe whatever you want to believe. You take the red pill, you stay in wonderland.'
LAURENCE FISHBURNE as Morpheus in *The Matrix*

How did it go?

Q   **I regularly suffer from nightmares – particularly about dying. Is there any remedy I can take for this?**

A   *A good one to try is aurum met. which is often used for depression. It's particularly suited to workaholics and those who set themselves high goals. A homeopath would also recommend going for long walks, relaxing and washing in cold water. If your nightmares started after a shock or trauma, try aconite.*

Q   **What can I expect from my first visit?**

A   *A first visit may last around an hour as the homeopath asks detailed questions to build a complete picture of you. As well as questions about any inherited problems, past illnesses, and diet, you may also be asked which side you sleep on, what type of weather you prefer and whether you have food preferences. Only then will the homeopath prescribe a remedy specifically to suit you.*

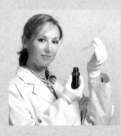

46

It makes scents

Oils, hot bath, aromatherapy candles – guaranteed to get you in the mood for bed.

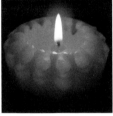

As you sink into a warm candlelit aromatherapy bath all the stresses of the day become a distant memory. Essential oils have the power to change the way you feel physically and emotionally — even some hospitals now use lavender oil to promote sleep.

Essential oils work on the central nervous system. When they're inhaled they affect the mood centres of your brain and when they're massaged onto your skin, they enter your bloodstream and cell tissues and are carried to every part of your body. They react with body chemistry in a way that's similar to drugs but slower and with fewer side effects. A lot of research has shown how oils can have a significant effect on our brain activity, alertness and moods. The right oils can relax the mind and body, control stress and relieve pain as well as beat insomnia – particularly when combined with massage.

Swap aromatherapy massages with your partner. Get him to lie comfortably on his front. Add a few drops of chamomile or rose into a light carrier oil, then dip your fingers in the oil. Place both your hands on the top of your partner's back near the shoulders, a few inches apart, then start stroking in a wide circular movement. Press into the upward stroke and glide back down, working your way down his back. Your arms will cross to make the circle so you should just lift one hand over the other to continue. Now for some kneading. Place both hands near his neck and shoulders with your fingers pointing away from you. Press into his body with the palm of one hand, pick up the flesh between your thumb and fingers and press it toward your resting hand. Release and repeat with the other hand. Alternate the circling and kneading for at least 15 minutes. Now it's your turn!

But for a quick and easy way to prepare your body for sleep, you can't beat an aromatherapy bath – put calming essential oils into a warm bath about 40 minutes before you go to bed. A fall in temperature is one of the triggers for sleep so you'll feel all warm and relaxed after a bath – then when your temperature drops 40 minutes later you'll be ready to shut down. Your bath should be warm enough to relax aching muscles and ease tension, but not too hot as this will make the oils evaporate more quickly.

THE OILS EVERY INSOMNIAC SHOULD OWN

Opt for oils that have a relaxing rather than invigorating aroma. Always dilute essential oils in a carrier oil such as sweet almond or grapeseed – with the exception of tea tree and lavender – as they'll burn your skin if applied neat. The ideal strength is five to six drops of essential oil to one tablespoon of carrier oil. Always do a patch test before massaging into your skin.

- Geranium. This oil strengthens the adrenal glands which work overtime when you're stressed. Combine with rosemary for maximum impact. For the best effect, add a few drops to your bath or listen to some music and put some drops in an oil burner.

- Lavender. It's the oil most often used for sleep problems as it helps reduce stress, anxiety and depression. Sprinkle a couple of drops on a tissue and inhale or, after a long, hard day put a few drops on your pillow to aid sleep.

- Frankincense. This oil is a great aphrodisiac if you want to get in the mood for sex. Have a bath together and add a few drops with sandalwood and a hint of jasmine to liven up your libido.

- Ylang ylang. This is also an aphrodisiac, but a sedative too so if the sex doesn't relax you the calming properties of this oil will. Add a couple of drops in a vaporiser for a soothing aroma.

- Chamomile. This calms the central nervous system and induces sleep. It's also a gentle antidepressant and stress reliever. Add a few drops of the oil to your bath.

Try another idea...

Essential oils are extracted from certain plants, flowers and herbs and are not taken internally. In herbalism, you take the very same plants in tea or as a pill. Find out more in IDEA 44, *Herb power*.

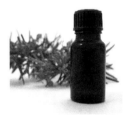

Defining idea...

'*There must be quite a few things that a hot bath won't cure, but I don't know many of them.*'

SYLVIA PLATH, *The Bell Jar*

Q **There's a big difference in price between essential oil makers – does this reflect their quality?**

A *Yes, most likely. Some have less pure oil so are unlikely to have much effect. Look for the words pure essential oil or look for oils with the Latin names of the plant on the label. Essential oils are like wine – you get good and bad years, and the price fluctuates from year to year. Colour is a good indicator of quality – avoid any oil that has a watery consistency, and always store them in a cool, dark place so they stay active.*

Q **Does it work straight away?**

A *Essential oils are not all absorbed into the body at the same rate. They can take 20 minutes or several hours depending on the oil and the individual body chemistry of the person being treated. On average oils take about 90 minutes to be absorbed. After several hours the oils leave your body. Regular treatments are needed to rebalance body systems and if you have been stressed or ill, it could take several weeks of treatment before you notice an improvement.*

Q **Why are oils blended together?**

A *Blending together changes the molecular structure of essential oils and when they're blended well it strengthens the effect. In general, oils from the same groups – citrus, floral, spicy and so on – and those which share similar constituents blend well.*

47

Get to the point

Sticking needles into you may not be the first thing you think of when trying to cure your sleep problems, but there's plenty of research to back it up.

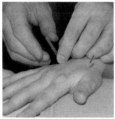

Acupuncture seems to have a calming effect on the nervous system and practitioners say it can help correct the imbalances causing insomnia — without any side effects.

Acupuncture, as I'm sure you know, involves inserting very fine needles into specific points on the surface of the body. These acupoints lie along channels of energy called meridians, which acupuncturists believe correspond to different inner organs. When these points are stimulated, it can trigger mental and physical changes – many of which can help your sleep problems.

Acupuncture has been shown to lower anxiety and increase levels of melatonin – your key sleep hormone. It also hikes the production of calming neurotransmitters such as serotonin and triggers endorphins in the brain that give you a greater sense of well-being. In one trial, 59% of people with insomnia had better sleep after

Here's an idea for you...

Try acupressure on the following points, using fingers instead of needles. Get close to the area and press in hard circular motions for up to three minutes. P6 – for relieving anxieties, particularly about relationships. It's two thumb widths above the crease of the wrist on the palm side of the forearm between the tendons in the centre of the arm. H7 – for calming an overactive mind. It's on the small finger side of the wrist crease in the hollow just below the bone near the outer edge of the wrist. P7 – to relax. It's on the inside of your wrist on the midpoint of the crease. GV24 – to relieve tension. It's half a thumb width above your hairline at the front of your head on the centre line. Having trouble finding the points? Shops now sell devices that find the point for you and produce small electrical impulses to stimulate it.

a daily acupuncture session for seven to ten days. In another study, people with sleep problems were fitted with a cone-shaped device (called an isocone) which massaged their 7 heart acupuncture points while they slept. They had more non-REM sleep so they slept for longer and woke up less during the night.

Acupuncturists believe that illness – including stress and insomnia – is caused by blockages in the flow of *chi* energy on the meridians so they will try to remove blockages and promote the flow of *chi* again. By inserting a needle or placing fingertip pressure on one of three hundred acupoints, they can fix any problems on a related meridian or body organ.

Acupuncturists often choose points on the heart or pericardium meridians to treat insomnia as these meridians are responsible for mental activity and consciousness. They'll choose many different combinations of points, however, depending on the cause of your insomnia – be it restless legs syndrome, headaches or any other pain that's keeping you up at night. Once they've selected your acupuncture points, the needles are quickly inserted – either by hand or through a guide tube. As few as 1 or 2 or as many as 20 or more needles may be used.

Of course, what you really want to know is, does it hurt? If done properly you shouldn't feel much when acupuncture needles are inserted – the needles are very fine and pass easily through the skin. You might get a dull or heavy feeling around the needle – this just means the treatment's working. The needles are usually left in for 15–30 minutes. And you'll probably need 6–10 treatments once a week before it works. Your relationship with your acupuncturist need not end there, however. Nearly everyone I know has an acupuncturist even though their original problem has been sorted – yes, needles are the new psycho-therapy. Regular maintenance sessions can keep your stress levels in check and stop your sleep problems coming back.

Make sure your acupuncturist is qualified and is a member of one the recognised professional bodies. Some medical doctors, nurses and physiotherapists also prac-tice acupuncture. But they may have done full acupuncture training or just a week-end course for a specific type of acupuncture such as pain relief. Always check qualifications and don't be afraid to ask about training and experience.

Still having trouble relieving stress? Try other alternative therapies that are good for stress – take a look at IDEA 44, *Herb power*, to find out about herbalism, and IDEA 46, *It makes scents*, for the lowdown on aromatherapy.

Try another idea…

'Anyone who can handle a needle convincingly makes us see a thread which is not there.'

Defining idea…

EH GOMBRICH, author

How did it go?

Q   **What happens in your first consultation?**

A   *The first thing the practitioner will do in a typical consultation is to take your pulse and check your tongue. Twelve pulses – including one for each internal organ – are felt along the radial artery on the outside of each wrist. The abdomen and certain acupuncture points may also be touched to check for tenderness or pain. The colour, shape and coating of your tongue, the face and skin are all checked for signs indicating which internal organs have problems.*

Q   **Can children be treated?**

A   *Yes, children and even babies respond very well to acupuncture. Treatment usually involves stimulation of the points by the fingers, by means of little 'rollers' or hand-held gadgets, or by quick insertion of small needles.*

Q   **Is there any risk of infection?**

A   *All properly trained acupuncturists follow rigorous hygiene and safety procedures to prevent any risk of infection to either their patients or themselves. The needles are sterilised to prevent any risk of infection and most now use disposable needles so that there's no risk of infection at all.*

48

Wakey wakey!

Alarm clock or not? The best option for a good night's sleep.

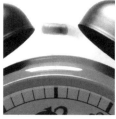

One minute you're fast asleep, the next you're leaping out of bed, your heart thumping. What woke you may sound like a fire bell, but it's only your alarm clock. You're awake, but still feel groggy. Is this really the best way to start the day?

If you wake up naturally, the light of dawn signals your body clock to release your wake-up hormones. An alarm clock obviously interferes with this natural process and allows you to wake up when it's convenient to you. OK, it may be masking the fact that you're not getting enough sleep, but the world would be thrown into chaos if we all woke up naturally. People would be wondering into offices at all times of the day – night owls, whose body clocks run slow, would probably get in the latest as they don't wake up naturally until late morning. And in the winter, everyone would turn up late because the sun rises much later and this delays the release of your wake-up hormones. In the summer, curtains protect us from the

Here's an idea for you... **Train yourself to wake up at a certain time – that way, the alarm won't seem so much of a shock. It's not that difficult to do. In fact you've probably done it yourself when you've had to get up for something important. Tell yourself the night before that you need to wake up at a certain time and after a few nights, it will happen.**

dawn light to prevent us from waking up at 5 in the morning but it's difficult to do anything in winter when it's pitch black outside.

SO WHAT CAN YOU DO?

You don't want to completely rely on an alarm clock – use one as an insurance policy in case you don't wake up in time. Ideally you should wake up just before your set time – that shows you've had enough sleep. Make sure the alarm clock you choose wakes you up how you want to. There's a lot of choice nowadays – so hunt around. Here are just a few I came across …

- A natural alarm clock. This simulates the sunrise and gradually becomes lighter and lighter over half an hour, so that you can wake up naturally whenever it suits you. This gradual lightening triggers your body to release all the wake-up hormones. The idea is you'll wake up more refreshed and in a better mood and have more energy all day. By putting your body clock in sync, the theory is you'll want to go to sleep earlier in the evening. There's normally a back-up-beeper for heavy sleepers and some even have a sunset go-to-sleep facility where the light slowly fades to darkness – ideal for young children or shift workers.
- Tailor-made alarm clock. These allow you to record your own wake-up sounds. Classical, jazz, rock … choose your favourite track of the moment. Or you can even record sounds – the sound of your children laughing perhaps or for some-

thing more surreal, your own voice telling you it's time to get up.

- Alarm clock with fade-in facility. The alarm or music gets gradually louder so you wake up more gently. Apparently, this makes it easier to remember your dreams.
- Talking alarm clock. One alarm clock I came across starts chatting to you after the alarm goes off. To turn it off you can say 'alarm off' or simply shake it. You can ask questions such as 'how do I look?' and the clock will give you a reply – either you look 'like a million dollars' or 'to tell you the truth – bleurgh!'
- Shaking alarm clock. Yes, this clock actually shakes the bed to wake you up. If that doesn't work, the flashing lights come on. Sounds like waking up to an erupting volcano to me, but it may work for you.

Work out how much sleep you need – if you're relying on an alarm clock you may not be getting enough. Check out IDEA 5, *Six, seven or eight?* and take the test.

Try another idea...

Whatever type you decide on, make sure you buy an alarm clock which allows you to dim the brightness of the LED display light. This light can disrupt your sleep and wake you up – particularly if you're a light sleeper and early in the morning when you spend more time in the lighter stages of sleep. Alternatively, turn your alarm clock away from you at night or use the alarm clock in your mobile phone.

'If you need an alarm clock to get up, you are sleep deprived.'

JAMES MAAS, sleep expert

Defining idea...

207

How did it go? **Q** **My journey to work is so erratic – sometimes it takes 20 minutes and other times over an hour so I have to set my alarm early just in case. When I get to work early, I just think about that extra time in bed I could have had. How can I squeeze in more sleep?**

A *There's not much you can do about that. If you're tired and really need that extra half an hour, you should think about going to bed half an hour earlier. In future, however, you may be able to get the extra sleep you need. A smart alarm clock that will allow you a lie-in or wake you up early depending on traffic conditions has been invented by British researchers. The clock has in-built internet access and retrieves relevant traffic information from across the web based on data you have given it, such as where you live, where you need to travel to and what time you need to arrive. The alarm clock will then work out what time you need to be woken. It's not available yet, but keep a look out – it soon will be.*

Q **I found it easy to train myself to wake up without an alarm clock. What's the mechanism at work here?**

A *Your unconscious mind now expects to wake up at a certain time. Your body ancipates the stress of waking up by releasing the stress hormone adrenocorticotropin.*

49

Wake-up stretches

This simple stretch routine will not only get your muscles ready for the day, it will also give you time to wake up properly, clear your head and lift your spirits.

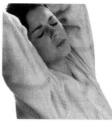

You have to get up, but you're convinced someone has attached lead weights to your limbs overnight. You're stiff, groggy and in a foul mood. And you know you're going to snap at the first person you encounter. Time to get moving, I think.

The following exercises will promote blood flow around your body, particularly to your extremities such as your feet, which receive less blood overnight. They're designed for every stage of the waking up process and you don't need to warm up. Start when you're still comfortably resting in your bed …

- *Still in bed.* While lying on your back, reach your arms over your head and straighten your legs, making yourself longer. Imagine you're being pulled in

Here's an idea for you... **Still need an extra boost even after those energy stretches? Why not brave a cold shower? Bathing in cold water can boost circulation and increase energy levels – take a three-minute hot shower followed by 40–60 seconds of cold water. Repeat three times if you dare.**

opposite directions; reach out your arms as far as you can, and push your legs as far as they'll go. If you're prone to calf cramps, keep your feet flexed. Hold this stretch for three deep breaths and release, letting your body relax into your bed.

- *Ready to get up.* Sit on the edge of your bed and slump your body over your legs. You should look like a rag doll bent at the waist. Starting from your lower back, slowly roll to a sitting position. To finish, slowly roll your shoulders back to correct posture – this should take 6 to 8 seconds – and look straight ahead. Just as slowly – again, taking 6 to 8 seconds – roll back down to the rag doll position, first tucking your head in to your chest, then rolling your shoulders forward, and finally curling down toward your knees.

- *Rise and shine.* Get out of bed then go on all fours on your bedroom floor and arch your back as high as possible. Repeat the arch movement slowly 12–15 times. This will release tension in the body and stretch out the muscles after a night's sleep.

- *Up and about.* Stand next to your bedroom wall for support, facing sideways, your feet about hip-width apart. Without bending your knees, slowly shift your weight to your toes, leaning slightly forward as far as you can without tipping or letting your heels come off the floor. Then shift your weight back to your heels, tilting backward without lifting your toes. Next, still keeping your feet flat on the floor, sway to the left and then to the right as far as possible. For more of a challenge, bring your feet closer together, and then try it with your eyes closed.

- *Time for the bends.* Go into your kitchen or dining room. Stand straight, holding a table or chair for balance. Take 3 seconds to bend your left knee, trying to get your calf as close to the back of your thigh as possible. Hold, then straighten your leg over 3 seconds. Repeat with your right leg.
- *Knees up Mother Brown.* Stand next to your kitchen or dining room wall for support and face sideways. Slowly raise your right knee over 3 seconds, bringing it as close to your chest as possible. Don't bend at the waist or hips. Hold for a second or two, then lower your leg over 3 seconds. Repeat with your left leg.
- *The ultimate energy kick.* Stand straight, holding your table or chair for support. Slowly lift your left leg 6 to 12 inches (15–30cm) to the side; do not bend your knee or upper body. Hold. Slowly lower, and repeat on your right side. Once you've mastered this, hold the table with one hand, then one finger, then no hands, then eyes closed.

All limbered up now? Why not enjoy one of the early morning bites in IDEA 50, *Breakfast boosters*, guaranteed to keep that spring in your step all morning.

Try another idea…

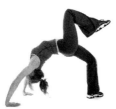

'I exercise every morning without fail. One eyelid goes up and the other follows.'
PETE POSTLETHWAITE, actor

Defining idea…

211

Q   **I like the sound of t'ai chi – would it help wake me up in the morning?**

A   It sure would. If it's good enough for the millions of Chinese and Japanese people who perform it every morning to prepare themselves for the day, then it'll probably be good for you too. This ancient Chinese practice incorporates strength training and flexibility work, and offers a moderate cardiovascular workout. Studies have shown that practising 20 minutes a day not only improves mood and energy levels, it also helps reduce stress levels and boosts your immune system. Other benefits? Better flexibility and posture, as well as improved circulation.

Q   **I sometimes wake up still tense after a night's sleep. What do you suggest?**

A   The stretches will help but you can also try a meridian massage, which will get your circulation going even if you don't believe in meridians (the pathways along which energy flows through the body). We can stimulate the flow of energy along the meridians by massaging in the direction of the energy flow. So using firm pressure, run both hands simultaneously down the outside of both legs, from thighs to ankles and in one flowing movement, back up the inside. Repeat several times. Starting from the back of the left hand and fingers, run the right palm up the back of the left arm and down the inside of the left arm. Finish the stroke with a flick of the right hand off the fingers of the left. Repeat several times, then work with the left hand on the right arm.

50

Breakfast boosters

A good breakfast prevents your energy levels from flagging and makes you brighter and happier. So why not set yourself up for the day with an early morning pick-me-up?

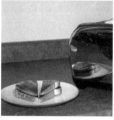

Do you rush out of the house in the morning without so much as a bite of toast? Well, don't be surprised if you're dozing at your desk by mid morning or you're unable to drag yourself off the sofa by mid afternoon.

Scientists have proved that the advice your mother gave you all those years ago was right: breakfast is the most important meal of the day. Yet about a fifth of us still skimp on early morning eating or skip breakfast altogether. Not only does missing breakfast leave you with low energy, it makes it harder for your body to get all the nutrients you need in a day. Breakfast can provide up to a quarter of your daily intake of certain vitamins and minerals – including vitamin C, which helps you drop off more easily at night, and the vital B vitamins that make your sleep hormones. There's also masses of research to show that eating a good breakfast means you're less likely to overeat for the rest of the day – particularly important in the evening when a big meal could disrupt your sleep.

Here's an idea for you... **Make your own muesli. Mix together a handful of oatflakes with your favourite dried fruits, nuts and shaved coconut. Add fruit and yoghurt to plain cereals or mix chopped nuts such as peanuts, hazelnuts or walnuts into porridge.**

TIME TO REFUEL

It's 7a.m., you've just woken up and the last thing you had to eat was a sandwich at 9p.m. What has your body been using to keep itself going for the last 10 hours without food? When you sleep, your metabolism slows down, but you still need a constant supply of energy in the form of glucose to keep your body, and particularly your brain, ticking over. Glucose is stored in your liver but, because it's not being replaced while you're asleep, your levels are pretty low when you wake up. Your brain needs a new supply to kickstart it into action again.

This is when breakfast performs its magic. By eating breakfast as soon as you can, you rev-up your metabolism and replenish the glucose you lost overnight, providing instant fuel for your brain to function throughout the day. Studies have shown that people who eat breakfast perform better mentally and verbally and concentrate better than those who don't. It can make us feel better about ourselves and boost energy for at least two hours – unlike a big lunch which can lead to an afternoon dip.

THE PERFECT COMBINATION

So what's the perfect breakfast? As well as making you more alert and giving you more energy, it should also keep you feeling fuller for longer. Go for a high-carbohydrate, low-fat meal with plenty of fibre, all washed down with a glass of orange or grapefruit juice or fruit tea. Good ones to try are:

- a bowl of fruit salad, topped with yoghurt and a good sprinkling of muesli
- a bowl of porridge, topped with chopped banana
- plain fat-free yoghurt with low-sugar muesli and mixed fresh berries
- one slice of wholegrain toast with fruit spread
- a bagel with low-fat cream cheese and pineapple slices
- two slices of wholemeal toast with marmite or peanut butter
- Shredded Wheat cereal with skimmed milk and a banana

If you're just not hungry when you get up, make sure you drink some milk, some fruit or vegetable juice or whizz up a tasty smoothie using milk and fresh, canned or frozen fruit. Something is better than nothing and you can have a sandwich, roll or some cheese and crackers later in the morning.

You've had breakfast and you're on top form. Check out IDEA 33, *Food for thought*, to make sure you're eating the right balance of foods to ensure a good night's sleep.

Try another idea…

'All happiness depends on a leisurely breakfast.'

JOHN GUNTHER, novelist

Defining idea…

How did it go?

Q **I love my fry-ups – fried eggs, bacon, fried bread, tomatoes, mushrooms, the works – all washed down with a sugary coffee. I do feel tired by about 10, though. What can I do to improve it?**

A   *Try a poached egg, toast and grilled bacon and tomatoes instead. It will slice off at least a third of the fat and nearly half the calories. Fruit juice is a healthier drink – it tastes sweet and its vitamin C content will also make it easier for your body to absorb iron from the rest of the breakfast. If you fancy an alternative blowout, why not try a 2-egg omelette made with low-fat cheese, chopped veggies and low-fat ham or turkey.*

Q **I'm just too busy in the morning to have breakfast. What can I do?**

A   *Nonsense. How long does it take to make toast or have a bowl of cereal? Before you get dressed pop some multigrain bread in the toaster and butter it afterwards. Or microwave a bowl of instant porridge as you pack your bag. Failing that, eat a banana or a breakfast bar. If you really have no time in the morning, make a breakfast the night before, which you can eat on the go – a bag of dried fruits and nuts and a bottle of fruit or vegetable juice, maybe, or wrap up some sticks of celery stuffed with peanut butter, pâté or soft cheese.*

Q **Does it matter which bread I have for my toast?**

A   *Choose wholemeal or wholewheat bread rather than white bread, because it takes longer to break down and stays in the stomach longer, keeping you feeling full. This means that you avoid mid-morning hunger pangs, so you're less likely to be tempted to snack on fatty and sugary snacks.*

51

The joy of zzzz

So you've adapted your sleep schedule, and your bedroom is a shrine to sleep – quiet, luxurious and free from clutter. Time for the pay-off – reaping the benefits of all the hard work you've put in.

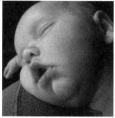

Twenty minutes before bed, you enjoy a banana and hot milky drink. After 15 minutes of yoga you crawl into bed and reach over to kiss your partner ...

A while later, in a post-coital glow, you drift off into a dreamless sleep and wake up after 8 hours feeling refreshed and regenerated. Add a few energy stretches and you're ready to meet the challenges of the day.

Once you're getting your full quota of sleep, you'll not only feel great but your health and well-being will be transformed too. Suddenly people will be saying all sorts of nice things to you.

Here's an idea for you…

Write down your recipe for good sleep. You'll have tried many things – some will have worked, others not. Make a list of everything that improved the quality of your sleep – from lavender essential oil in your bath to visualising a relaxing beach scene. If you start getting sleepless nights again or start slacking on your new schedule, you can refer to your notes.

■ *'You look really well.'* It's not called beauty sleep for nothing! You can spend a fortune on expensive skin creams and watch your diet, but you need your sleep for youthful-looking skin. Our body clock determines when certain body cells are most active – and our skin cells repair themselves more effectively at night. Research shows that cell regeneration more than doubles overnight and is most active between 11p. m. and 4a.m. Production of collagen – the skin's natural support structure which is vital for keeping skin smooth, supple and youthful – is also boosted. And harmful free radicals – rogue cell-destroying molecules which can lead to premature ageing – are scavenged and cell damage is repaired. And what about those dark circles around the eyes you've been sporting for the last few months? A thing of the past.

■ *'Hey, you're in a good mood.'* You've probably been a bit cranky and antisocial recently, but now you're getting enough sleep you're back on form. Many of the neurotransmitters in the brain that regulate sleep also regulate mood, which is why sleep deprivation is associated with mood swings. Neurotransmitters, which carry messages to the brain, get sluggish along the way and need to be replenished during sleep. When they are, your spirits will be high.

- *'You don't seem so stressed any more.'* Your permanent frown has disappeared. You're in the habit of writing down your worries – and possible solutions – at least once a week so you don't go to bed with a suitcase full of concerns. And because you're getting a good night's sleep you're better able to cope with everyday events so you don't get so affected by stress.

'Sleep is that golden chain that ties health and our bodies together.'
THOMAS DEKKER, playwright
(1577-1632)

 Defining idea...

- *'Have you lost weight?'* If you're getting enough sleep now, your appetite will be back to normal. Sleep loss interferes with the secretion of cortisol, a hormone that regulates appetite. So when your cortisol levels were out of whack, you were probably feeling hungry even if you'd had enough to eat. Carbohydrates also metabolise slower when you're sleep deprived, causing sugars to linger in the blood and jack up insulin production, which increases the storage of body fat.

- *'You haven't had a cold for ages.'* Gone are the days of waking up next to a mountain of tissues. Sleep helps your body fight infection because your immune system releases a sleep-inducing chemical while fighting a cold or an infection. Sleep also helps the body conserve energy and other resources that the immune system needs to mount an effective attack.

- *'Wow! You were sharp in that meeting.'* Now that you're sleeping, you'll be able to concentrate on what people are saying, your memory has returned and you can think more clearly.

If you've still got any queries try IDEA 52, *Quirky questions*. It's got every silly thing you wanted to know about sleep but had no one to ask.

 Try another idea...

219

How did it go?

Q **I'm waking up refreshed for the first time in ages. But why am I not dreaming any more?**

A *You'll still be having REM sleep, which is when you dream – it's just that you're now sleeping more deeply and are less likely to wake up in the night. You're more likely to remember your dreams if your sleep is being interrupted.*

Q **I'm sleeping well now, but how can I stop myself slipping back into old ways again?**

A *If you stick to the rules, you should be OK. Everyone has the odd sleepless night – it's part of being human – you just need to make sure it doesn't turn into a habit again. So keep up your relaxing bedtime ritual, get plenty of exercise in the day and cut down on stimulants like caffeine and alcohol. Never bring your worries to bed with you – work out how you're going to deal with them earlier in the day. And if insomnia returns only go to bed when you're tired and if you can't fall asleep after 20 minutes get out of bed and do something relaxing before returning to bed. Remember your bedroom is for sleep and sex only.*

Q **I feel full of energy and completely alert in the day since sorting my sleep problems. I'm only getting 7 hours of sleep a night though – should I be having more?**

A *It's a myth that we need 8 hours of sleep a night. If 7 hours – or even less – works for you, that's fine.*

52

Quirky questions

Can you sleep with your eyes open? This and other quirky questions answered.

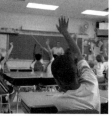

Okay it may be sleep trivia, but it's still worth knowing. Here are the answers to all those niggling questions that everyone's wanted to know about sleep but didn't know who to ask.

- *Do people sleep significantly longer when they're not working?*

On average people sleep for just 6.7 hours before a working day and 7.1 hours before a day off. One in six adults say they would use their holidays to make up the sleep they do not get in their day-to-day lives.

- *Do people bother to catch up on sleep?*

Of those who fall short on their sleep needs, women are more likely to catch up by having an early night during the week. Men favour a lie-in at weekends.

Ask your friends what position they sleep in – apparently this reveals something about the kind of person they are. If they curl up in the foetus position – the most common sleeping position – they're tough on the outside but sensitive at heart. But lying on their side with both arms down by their side means they're easy going and sociable. If they sleep on their side with both arms out in front they're said to have an open nature, but can be suspicious and cynical. Do they lie on their back with both arms pinned to their sides? They're quiet and reserved with high standards. If they lie on their back with both arms up around the pillow, they'll make a good friend because they're always ready to listen to others, and offer help when needed. If they lie on their front with their hands around the pillow and their head turned to one side, they're likely to be gregarious, but sensitive to criticism.

■ *What's the longest amount of time someone has gone without sleep?*

The record is 18 days, 21 hours, 40 minutes after which the record holder reported hallucinations, paranoia, blurred vision, slurred speech and memory and concentration lapses.

■ *How loud is the loudest snore?*

One British snoring champion had a 92 decibel snore – louder than a pneumatic drill. Needless to say, his long-suffering wife is deaf in one ear.

■ *Can you sleep with your eyes open?*

Yes. Many parents claim their babies sleep with their eyes open or partially open. Adults can take cat naps with their eyes open without being aware of it and sleepwalkers are technically asleep even though they have their eyes open and appear to be awake. Incidentally, fish cannot close their eyes because they don't have eyelids. It is controversial as to whether fish sleep at all.

■ *Do we sleep longer than other animals?*

Humans sleep on average around three hours less than other primates like chimps, rhesus monkeys, squirrel monkeys and baboons, all of whom sleep for 10 hours.

If you want to find out more about the significance of your dreams and how to make them work for you, check out IDEA 28, *Dreamworks*.

Try another idea...

■ *Can you sleep standing up?*

No – you'd fall down as soon as your muscles relaxed. To stay standing you have to keep certain muscles tense, and to control these muscles you have to be conscious. When you fall asleep, you become unconscious so can't stay standing. Some animals can, however. Horses, for instance, have a system of tendons and ligaments that hold them in the standing position while their muscles relax. So they can lie down or stand up to sleep.

■ *How long do dreams last?*

Most dreams last as long as REM sleep – about 20 minutes each. And they're in real time – that means if you're dreaming about having a bath it's going to take about the same time as it does in real life. With the more surreal dreams it's more difficult to estimate – how long does it take to fly to work on a magic carpet?

'If there are no stupid questions, then what kind of questions do stupid people ask? Do they get smart just in time to ask questions?'
SCOTT ADAMS, US cartoonist

Defining idea...

■ *Do we dream in colour?*

Dreams usually start in colour, but the image soon fades into black and white.

■ *Is it possible not to dream?*

Most people dream, but just don't remember them. Drug treatments for people with depression often knock out dream sleep. This is because they tend to have sad and miserable dreams which may lead to more sad thoughts the next day. Patients treated this way have little or no dreaming sleep while they're taking antidepressants. Their mental health improves and there are no bad psychological side effects such as loss of memory. This shows that dream sleep may not be so critical to memory as some people have previously thought.

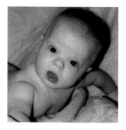

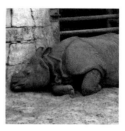

Q **Recently I dreamed that there was a stranger in my room and I was sitting up in my bed, frozen with fear unable to move. Then I woke up and was actually sitting in my bed.**

How did it go?

A *You could have been experiencing sleep paralysis. This is when you wake up from a dream and find that you cannot move. It can be particularly frightening if you're dreaming that someone's in the room or there's a burglar in the house. You may even try in vain to cry out. These episodes can last from a few seconds to a few minutes. It happens because the line between being awake and REM sleep has been blurred. Your brain's awake but you're still experiencing the paralysis of REM sleep. Sleep paralysis is not dangerous, however. It's normally associated with narcolepsy but you can get it if you're very sleep deprived, too.*

Q **Am I taller when I wake up than when I go to sleep?**

A *Yes. This is because the discs in your spine are hydrophilic, which means they suck up water while you sleep when there's no pressure on them. After getting up, the pressure of walking around and using your muscles compress your spine and the fluid is squeezed out. You're not going to wake up the height of a catwalk model, but ...*

Q **Will a loud noise influence my dreams?**

A *Probably not. Your alarm clock rings and you wake up to memories of a fire breaking out, fire engines arriving with sirens blasting. Because the alarm is still ringing, it's easy to think the sound triggered the dream. But all it does is pluck a previous scene from your dream or memory.*

225

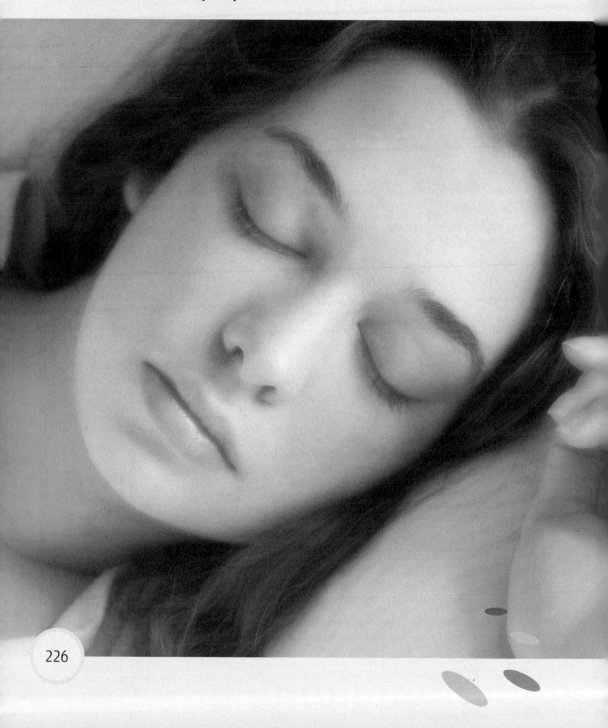

The end ...

Or is it a new beginning?

We hope that the ideas in this book will have inspired you to try some new ways to feel rested and refreshed. We hope you've found that making small but effective lifestyle changes has worked and that you're already turning your bedroom into a sleep sanctuary, practising yoga and stocking your fridge with sleep-inducing snacks. You should be well on your way to a healthier, more alert and happier you, bursting with vitality.

So, why not let *us* know all about it? Tell us how you got on. What did it for you – what really helped you to drift off and sleep well every night? Maybe you've got some tips of your own you want to share (see next page if so). And if you liked this book you may find we have even more brilliant ideas that could change other areas of your life for the better.

You'll find the Infinite Ideas crew waiting for you online at www.infideas.com.

Or if you prefer to write, then send your letters to:
Sleep Deep
The Infinite Ideas Company Ltd
36 St Giles, Oxford OX1 3LD, United Kingdom

We want to know what you think, because we're all working on making our lives better too. Give us your feedback and you could win a copy of another *52 Brilliant Ideas* book of your choice. Or maybe get a crack at writing your own.

Good luck. Be brilliant.

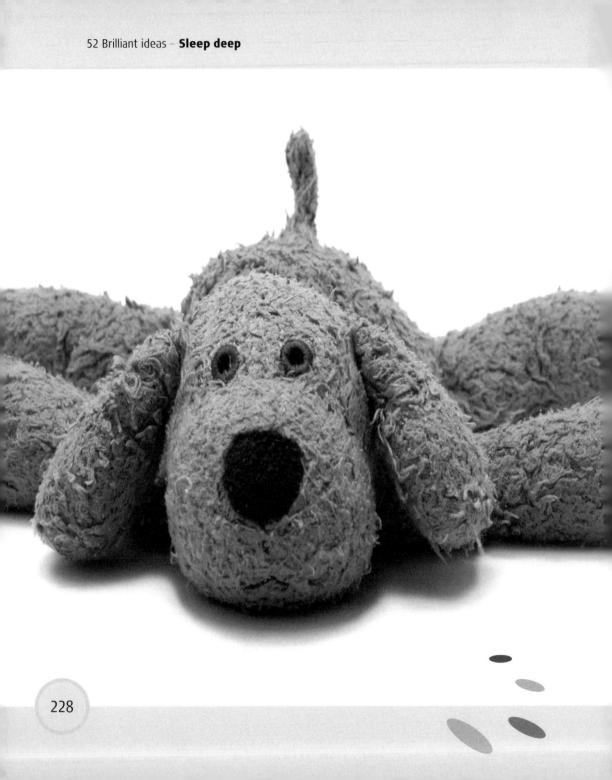

Offer one

CASH IN YOUR IDEAS

We hope you enjoy this book. We hope it inspires, amuses, educates and entertains you. But we don't assume that you're a novice, or that this is the first book that you've bought on the subject. You've got ideas of your own. Maybe our author has missed an idea that you use successfully. If so, why not send it to us by e-mail: yourauthormissedatrick@infideas.com, and if we like it we'll post it on our bulletin board. Better still, if your idea makes it into print we'll send you four books of your choice, or the cash equivalent. You'll be fully credited so that everyone knows you've had another Brilliant Idea.

Offer two

HOW COULD YOU REFUSE?

Amazing discounts on bulk quantities of Infinite Ideas books are available to corporations, professional associations and other organisations.

For details call us on:
+44 (0)1865 514888
fax: +44 (0)1865 514777
or e-mail: info@infideas.com

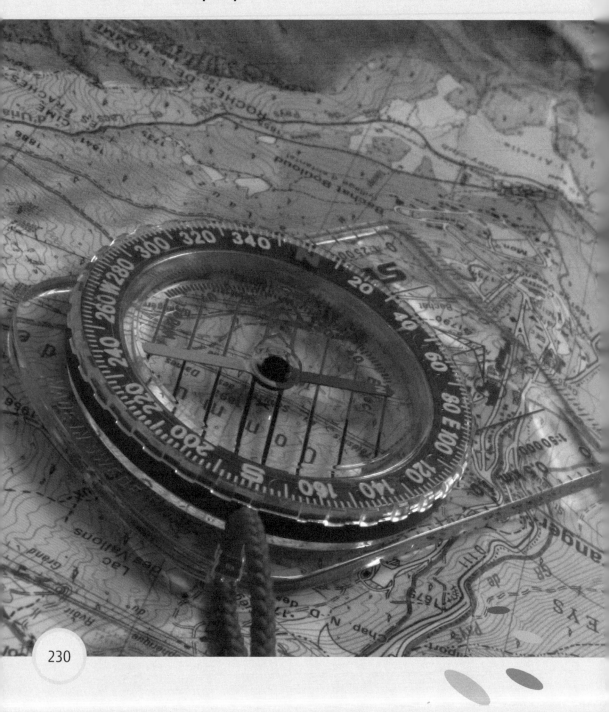

Where it's at ...

Even more brilliant ideas ...

Live longer
Sally Brown

"You can live a long and healthy life. Amazingly, anti-ageing scientists believe that only 1 in 10,000 people die of old age. The vast majority of us die prematurely from what we've come to call 'natural causes'. In fact, cell structure studies show that biologically our true lifespan is between 110 and 120 years!

All the advice you'll find in Live longer is achievable and can be fun too! Some of the best anti-ageing strategies involve having sex, drinking red wine and spending time with friends. So, live long and enjoy!" – **Sally Brown**

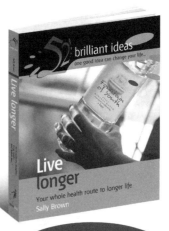

Look gorgeous always
Linda Bird

"Looking beautiful is about much more than possessing fantastic cheek-bones and endless legs, though of course, great genes do help. The good news is that vitality, confidence, a savvy wardrobe, a few great make up and grooming tricks can work wonders too."

"The trick is to look after yourself, and to learn how to use what you've got to your best advantage. It's about maximising your beautiful bits, minimising the less beautiful ones, and faking a few more. "

"Look gorgeous always will help you unlock the ravishing creature that lies within. It provides lots of simple but ingenious tips that that I've learned from the leading lights in health and beauty. Try these brilliant ideas today – and feel more gorgeous, instantly!" – **Linda Bird**

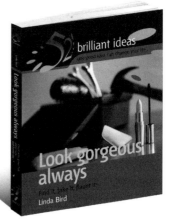

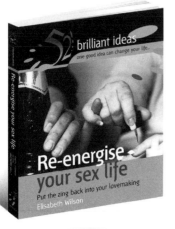

Re-energise your sex life

Elisabeth Wilson

"Sex manuals. They're either full of photos of impossibly lithesome twenty-somethings doing it in a state of almost clinical cleanliness or line drawings of men with beards who look like they're straight out of a Bee Gees tribute band."

"Well, this isn't a sex manual. You won't find any pictures in here. What you will find is inspirational ideas for people who've lost a little of that zing. So if you and your partner are in a bit of a rut, too tired from work or from looking after the kids to even feign headaches let alone orgasms, then I can help!" – **Elisabeth Wilson**

Available from all good bookshops and online at www.amazon.co.uk

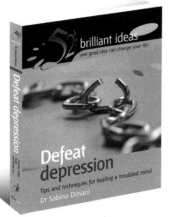

Defeat depression

Sabrina Dosani

"It is reckoned an average of 1 out of 18 people suffers from depression, and that it costs the economy in the region of 9 billion pounds per annum both in treatment and in lost work days. And yet, most people don't really understand what depression is and many of the symptoms that accompany it."

"This is a subject I'm absolutely passionate about. When I was a medical student, I became depressed and ended up in hospital myself. I learned a lot and can vouch for all the ideas in this book, having seen them work for either myself or my patients." – **Dr Sabina Dosani**